ESSENTIAL SKILLS IN FAMILY THERAPY

THE GUILFORD FAMILY THERAPY SERIES
Michael P. Nichols, Series Editor

ESSENTIAL SKILLS
IN FAMILY THERAPY

*From the First Interview
to Termination*

SECOND EDITION

JoEllen Patterson
Lee Williams
Todd M. Edwards
Larry Chamow
Claudia Grauf-Grounds

Foreword by Douglas H. Sprenkle

THE GUILFORD PRESS
New York   London

© 2009 The Guilford Press
A Division of Guilford Publications, Inc.
72 Spring Street, New York, NY 10012
www.guilford.com

Printed in the United States of America

This book is printed on acid-free paper.

Last digit is print number: 9   8   7   6   5   4   3   2   1

The authors have checked with sources believed to be reliable in
their efforts to provide information that is complete and generally
in accord with the standards of practice that are accepted at the time
of publication. However, in view of the possibility of human error or
changes in medical sciences, neither the authors, nor the editor and
publisher, nor any other party who has been involved in the preparation
or publication of this work warrants that the information contained
herein is in every respect accurate or complete, and they are not
responsible for any errors or omissions or the results obtained from
the use of such information. Readers are encouraged to confirm the
information contained in this book with other sources.

Library of Congress Cataloging-in-Publication Data

Essential skills in family therapy : from the first interview to termination
  / JoEllen Patterson ... [et al.] ; with foreword by Douglas H. Sprenkle.
  — 2nd ed.
    p. cm. — (The Guilford family therapy series)
  Includes bibliographical references and index.
  ISBN 978-1-60623-305-4 (hardcover : alk. paper)
  1. Family psychotherapy.   2. Family psychotherapy—
Practice.   I. Patterson, JoEllen.
  RC488.5.E79 2009
  616.89′156—dc22
                                            2009016133

In memory of George Sargent, PhD,
our friend, mentor, and colleague

About the Authors

JoEllen Patterson, PhD, is Professor of Marital and Family Therapy at the University of San Diego and Associate Clinical Professor in the Department of Family and Preventive Medicine and the Department of Psychiatry at the University of California, San Diego. She has written several books and numerous articles on family therapy training and the integration of mental health services into primary care.

Lee Williams, PhD, is Professor of Marital and Family Therapy at the University of San Diego and does couple therapy with veterans at the VA San Diego Medical Center. He has conducted research and published several articles on marriage preparation, interchurch couples, and family therapy training.

Todd M. Edwards, PhD, is Associate Professor and Director of the Marital and Family Therapy Program at the University of San Diego. He is a practicing family therapist and serves as Assistant Clinical Professor in the Department of Family and Preventive Medicine at the University of California, San Diego. His primary clinical and research interests are collaboration between family therapists and medical professionals, medical family therapy, and medical family therapy training.

Larry Chamow, PhD, is Clinical Professor of Marital and Family Therapy at the University of San Diego and is in full-time private practice at the Pacific Family Institute in Carlsbad, California. His interests and publications focus on couple therapy, supervision, the self of the therapist, and family businesses.

Claudia Grauf-Grounds, PhD, is Professor and Chair of Marriage and Family Therapy at Seattle Pacific University and a clinical faculty member at the University of Washington School of Medicine. She conducts research, publishes, and presents on family therapy training and collaborative healthcare models, including spirituality. She has been honored as Supervisor of the Year by the Washington Association for Marriage and Family Therapy.

Acknowledgments

This book is a joint effort of the authors and reflects conversations we have had at the University of San Diego over the last 10 years. Our editor at The Guilford Press, Jim Nageotte, inspired us to share our best ideas. Emily Ferguson, our graduate assistant/editor/reviewer, kept us on track and attended to the many details that we might have overlooked. Our students continue to challenge us to find new ways to teach family therapy. Finally, we are most grateful to our own families and the inspiration they provide for our work.

Foreword

JoEllen Patterson, Lee Williams, Todd Edwards, Larry Chamow, and Claudia Grauf-Grounds have done it again! When I wrote the foreword to the first edition of this book in 1998, I predicted it would become the "benchmark volume for beginning therapists." I am confident that the plaudits the book received during the past decade will resound for at least another 10 years with the publication of this new version. It is remarkable that in a relatively brief volume Patterson et al. spell out the day-to-day issues facing the beginning therapist so comprehensively as well as sensitively. Now an expanded and revised edition adds "up-to-date" to the adjectives that describe what my colleagues and I consider a gem within the training literature.

The authors took the strengths of the first edition and embellished them. First, their approach is biopsychosocial. Although it is principally a book about learning systemic therapy and appreciating the great contributions of this paradigm, this volume is written in dialogue with the many other disciplines and approaches to mental health about which the beginning therapist must be familiar. The authors wisely take the position that family therapy is not an isolated "cure-all," and they avoid the hubris that has marked some of the more extreme presentations of systemic therapy. As with the first edition, there is attention to DSM diagnoses and mental illness; however, the new volume provides important updates on psychotic disorders, mood disorders, anxiety, and substance abuse, as well as new information on topics like somatizing disorders and impulse control disorders. There are also new sections on evidence-based medicine, genetics, and neuroscience. To the authors' credit, the beginning therapist learns about systemic therapy in the larger context of healthcare delivery.

Second, the volume is a marvelous resource of training materials on such topics as informed consent; release of information; assessing for suicidality, substance abuse, violence, and duty-to-warn issues; and the basics of pharmacology and referral. Most of these topics have been substantially revised and updated, and the book also contains highly valuable forms, tables, and checklists that greatly facilitate learning.

Third, the book proceeds chronologically from first thoughts about doing therapy (and managing anxiety and confidence), through initial interviews, midtherapy, and on to a thoughtful chapter on termination. This chapter now includes expanded guidelines on transferring cases and the needs of the client being transferred, as well as the concerns of the outgoing and incoming therapist. I have never seen these issues addressed before and found the discussion useful even as a very experienced therapist/supervisor.

Fourth, the volume pays considerable attention to self-of-the-therapist issues that many of us consider invaluable for beginning therapists. In the second edition, the theme of therapist development is emphasized in the first chapter and addressed throughout the volume. Topics like therapist burnout, an expanded section on therapist reluctance to intervene, and a new and creative section on dealing with clients we dislike are part of this emphasis.

Fifth, and close to my heart as a common factors scholar, the volume takes an integrative approach to the therapeutic enterprise. You can benefit from this book regardless of your theoretical orientation since the authors focus on conceptualizations and interventions that cut across the major models of family therapy. As examples, Chapter 5, "Developing a Treatment Focus," a chapter on case conceptualization, is highly integrative. Chapter 6 contains a section on "Interventions Unique to the Systemic Family Therapist" that emphasizes core interventions that virtually all systemic therapists practice regardless of theoretical orientation. Chapter 8, on couple therapy, contains seven key principles for doing couple therapy that I believe would be just as useful to therapists with approaches as diverse as solution focused, object relations, or emotion focused. I believe this is a wise strategy by the authors since many family therapy models emphasize similar change mechanisms even though they are couched in different language and specific techniques. Furthermore, advocates of the various models notwithstanding, there is almost no empirical evidence for the relative efficacy of one family therapy model over other credible family therapy models.

Sixth, the book deals with important training issues like the role of supervision in the development of beginning therapists. The new edition stresses challenges that can come from having multiple supervisors and the problems that arise when there is a questionable fit between trainee and supervisor. In the strong Chapter 10, on getting unstuck, students are taught how to do a technology-based literature search on client problems, how to evaluate Internet resources, and how to evaluate empirical literature generally. Throughout the volume, cutting-edge training issues are addressed, such as how to do motivational interviewing and how to match interventions with the stage of change of the client.

As I said in my foreword to the first volume, "Reading and digesting this book may help the novice to feel like he/she is carrying with him/her a wise and compassionate supervisor." To those adjectives I would add the word "trustworthy." Having taught family therapy for 36 years, and having edited a major journal, while I am by no means an expert on everything, I know many areas well enough to recognize when authors speak with credibility and authority. I trust this author team and so, I believe, can you. If you are an experienced therapist/supervisor, you will find yourself saying, "I wish I had written this book." If you are the target audience, the beginning therapist, you will say, *"Essential Skills in Family Therapy* empowered me to do my best work."

DOUGLAS H. SPRENKLE, PhD
Department of Child Development
and Family Studies
Purdue University

Preface

More than a decade ago, we wrote *Essential Skills in Family Therapy* for our students at the University of San Diego (USD). We hoped that other family therapy students would find the information in it useful, but we wrote the book as if it were a personal letter to our students. Our letter attempted to answer the questions our students most frequently asked and also to answer some questions we thought they wanted to ask. For example, our students commonly reported feeling inadequate during the first few months of their clinical work. Other students had concerns about loyalty. If they found value in an individual treatment model, could they still be family therapists? As they advanced in their training, their questions became more complex. For example, they wondered how to balance individual, couple, and family assessment. They considered the impact of psychotropic medications on their clients and how they could coordinate care with physicians.

A strength and a weakness of our program has been that USD does not have its own training clinic. Thus, from their first clinical days, our students see clients in community settings where the focus is on expedient, cost-effective treatments. In addition, our students work with a variety of professionals including physicians, attorneys, school counselors, teachers, and other mental health professionals. While we struggle with gently easing our students into their roles as therapists, we also recognize that the community clinics' focus on results translates into a training emphasis at USD on what works, regardless of the treatments' origins.

Together, the USD faculty has developed some core beliefs that have guided our program. Following the tenets of George Engel, we believe a biopsychosocial perspective should guide our work, while placing particular emphasis on systemic thinking. In addition, we believe that our primary goal is to help individual clients and their families, and we are open to all ideas, procedures, treatments, and models that help us achieve that goal. Finally, regardless of the treatment, we believe that clients are strengthened when therapists can enlist family members in caring for each other. These tenets have continued to guide our work for the last 10 years.

Essential Skills in Family Therapy reflects the USD program's focus on students, its pragmatic approach to treatment, its regard for multidisciplinary perspectives, and its respect for the influence of families on clients. Since we wrote the first edition, these beliefs have guided us, and we've simultaneously evolved. This second edition reflects the new influences that have begun to shape our teaching and our clinical work. We've tried to mention most of the significant, new influences on our work. But we found that putting all of the new information in one book that is meant to be a concise introduction became untenable. Thus, we've written two other books for The Guilford Press that we hope augment the core ideas introduced in this volume: *The Therapist's Guide to Psychopharmacology* by Patterson, Albala, McCahill, and Edwards (2006) discusses strategies for providing cotreatment with physicians and highlights the importance of families in medication decision making and involvement in treatment. In addition, as *Essential Skills* goes to press, we are working on a companion volume that will provide the beginning therapist with more extensive instruction on assessment. The forthcoming book will build and expand upon the ideas found in Chapter 4 on assessment.

During the past 10 years, we have been heartened to learn that students in the United States and abroad have found this book both practical and clear. Our goal has been to condense the many ideas and models that we've learned into a succinct practical guide. We hope that the second edition of *Essential Skills* reflects our purpose.

Contents

CHAPTER 1

The Beginning Family Therapist

Taking On the Challenge

Tom is handed the intake paperwork for his first client at his new practicum site. Both excited and anxious, he scans the information. In the section on "primary reason for coming to therapy," the client has written, "Need ways to cope with my husband's drinking and his hitting the children." Tom grows more apprehensive as he wonders where to start. Should he simply listen to the woman's story as it unfolds? Or should he take a more direct approach and immediately assess for a substance abuse problem? Still another focus is the indication of child abuse. Perhaps this very serious matter takes precedence over every other issue.

Sally reviews today's back-to-back schedule and wonders if she will make it through the day. After learning yesterday that her father has cancer and is likely to die within the year, she tossed and turned all night. Exhausted but wanting to do a good job with her clients, she begins thinking about her first client family that day. The Joneses have an 8-year-old son with a multitude of problems: leukemia and attention-deficit/hyperactivity disorder, to name two. He has been referred by the family's physician "to develop coping skills." For a fleeting moment, Sally wonders if the pain she feels about her father will affect her therapy today, but she does not have much time to reflect on this question because her first session starts in 5 minutes.

Ann winces as she recalls her group supervision session yesterday. She had thought the videotaped session of her work with Mrs. Thomas showed what excellent joining skills she had. It would be clear to her supervisor and her fellow students that Mrs. Thomas liked therapy and took Ann's suggestions very seriously. But instead of focusing on the therapist–client rapport, the group had overwhelmed Ann with assessment questions she had not even considered. How was Mrs. Thomas's divorce connected to her depression? Did Ann think her late-night alcohol use reflected a substance abuse problem? Were Mrs. Thomas's children being neglected because she had little energy or time for parenting? What should Ann's level of involvement be in helping Mrs. Thomas find a job? Ann wondered if she had the necessary qualities to even be the therapist when she had so clearly missed important assessment questions for her client.

Most beginning therapists experience a host of anxious feelings when they start clinical work (Skovholt & Rønnestad, 2003). They are aware of their inadequacies more than their strengths, and need help to learn how to acquire the skills, knowledge, and sense of competency necessary to do good clinical work.

Many therapists complete the didactic part of their training with a sense of mastery and competence. After all, by the time they enter graduate school, the life of a student is very familiar, and they are accustomed to academic achievement in their course work. Academic accomplishments, however, do not necessarily translate easily into therapeutic competence. Faculty and students are left wondering how best to impart and acquire, respectively, the skills basic to clinical work.

The gap between academic work and the implementation of techniques or the application of theories in clinical sessions can seem huge. After a year of intense academic instruction, students often begin their clinical work with unstated questions:

"What am I supposed to say to the client?"

"How do I handle situation X?"

"What should happen after I complete the intake form?"

"Can clients tell I'm new at this and feeling completely inadequate and overwhelmed?"

"How do I keep all the information from the session clear and how do I know what is most important?"

"If I don't use a powerful intervention or technique during the first couple of sessions, am I a failure?"

"I know I should have a theory for this case, but I just don't understand how to apply information from my theories class to this acting-out adolescent and her hostile mother."

"How will I know if the clients actually get better?"

What students need is a way to develop their skills as therapists as they begin their clinical work. This book provides practical, "how to" guidelines on essential therapeutic skills from thorough assessment to careful treatment planning, from the nuts and bolts of specific interventions to the nuances of establishing therapeutic relationships and troubleshooting when treatment gets "stuck."

Reflecting the trend toward integrative approaches in family therapy, mental health, and the medical field, we stress a biopsychosocial view of assessment and treatment. This perspective provides the clinician an effective and comprehensive framework for addressing the broad issues that clients can present in therapy. Thus, while family interaction remains a focus of attention herein, our goal is to prepare beginning therapists to integrate information and skills from other areas as well to best meet the needs of diverse client families.

The ability to integrate family therapy theory and interventions with individual diagnosis and treatment will be especially valuable as therapists begin their careers. While family therapy offers a unique and important perspective in clinical work, much of what goes on in treatment shares common assumptions with all therapies. Certain clinical skills—assessing for suicide risk or substance abuse, making an effective referral—are intrinsic to any good therapy. This book goes beyond the boundaries of traditional family therapy to be as inclusive as possible of essential clinical skills.

Frequently, beginning family therapy students make treatment decisions based on their supervisors' favorite theoretical orientation or the specific theoretical approach predominant in their clinic. We believe that assessing the appropriateness of a family therapy treatment for a specific problem is an essential clinical skill. It is important to be able to recognize when a problem is outside the scope of a family therapist's practice (or skill level) and could best be treated by another mental health professional or in tandem with another healthcare professional.

Indeed, research on biological etiologies of mental illness and psychopharmacology suggests that therapists must be conversant with more than "talk therapies." A growing focus on treatment teams and multidisciplinary treatment approaches means that therapists must increasingly attend to the biological component of the biopsychosocial model and learn to collaborate with other healthcare professionals. A knowledge base in medication management and the ability to consult with physicians is one aspect of this multidisciplinary approach.

While the bulk of this book discusses specific processes and skills that are important throughout the therapeutic journey, we devote the first chapter to that most basic of concerns for the beginning therapist—understanding and managing beginners' jitters.

GETTING STARTED

> "It was my first session with a client and my heart was racing. I had no idea what to do with this family, and I wasn't really sure if they knew why they were all there. I was talking with the mother, who requested the appointment, to find out how much the other family members knew about why they came in when I realized that I didn't really like this lady.... "

This story, shared by a practicum student, encompasses two essential and pressing issues shared by most beginning therapists. One revolves around the question "What do I do?" and the other involves managing one's own feelings and reactions to diverse clients and clinical situations.

Learning the art and science of doing therapy is a challenging task, particularly when first seeing clients. Many beginning therapists have periodic feelings of inadequacy and insecurity about their clinical abilities. Some may fear that they will directly harm their clients or cause their conditions to deteriorate because of clinical mistakes. Others fear that they will not be able to help their clients because of their inexperience. A few doubt their talent and ability as therapists to the extent that they seriously question whether to remain in the field.

Therapists and supervisors alike need to see confidence issues from a developmental perspective (Bischoff & Barton, 2002). Given their lack of clinical experience, it is only natural that beginning therapists question their competence. In fact, as supervisors, we worry more about beginning therapists who seem extremely confident in their abilities. This feeling of confidence is incongruent with the complexity and difficulty of learning to do therapy well.

MANAGING ANXIETY AND ISSUES
OF CONFIDENCE

How does the beginning therapist deal with a lack of confidence, or with feeling overwhelmed and anxious? First, therapists must recognize that these feelings are completely normal. Although the intensity of the feelings and the way of coping will vary from therapist to therapist, every beginning therapist struggles to some degree with these feelings. Therapists who do not acknowledge this often get trapped in a vicious circle. They interpret feelings of being overwhelmed as a possible sign that they are not cut out to be therapists, which only serves to fuel their anxiety.

Second, beginning therapists need to share these experiences with other therapists and supervisors. Sharing feelings of anxiety or lack of confidence can help to normalize the experience. Unfortunately, it is fear of being incompetent or a failure that prevents beginning therapists from sharing their struggles with others. When a therapist does take the risk and shares his or her fears with peers, others generally disclose the same worries. This in turn helps the beginning therapist to accept that these struggles are developmentally appropriate rather than a sign of being unsuited for the profession.

Third, distorted cognitions or beliefs may contribute to a therapist's fears or struggles with confidence. These can be addressed using cognitive restructuring. The first step is for the therapist to identify cognitions or beliefs about the ability to do therapy effectively. For example, some beginners have questioned the ethicality of treating difficult clients (or any client at all!) when more experienced therapists are available. When distortions are identified, perhaps with a supervisor's help, they can be "replaced" with more constructive thoughts that benefit coping and decrease anxiety. Recalling that such seasoned clinicians as Salvador Minuchin and Virginia Satir were once beginners can also help. A good battery of constructive thoughts and images goes a long way toward soothing beginners' jitters.

Fourth, it is crucial to realize that the therapist–client relationship is inherently therapeutic. A therapist doesn't need to *do* something for clients to have a positive experience. This is very reassuring to most beginning therapists because they generally have confidence in their relational skills. When beginning therapists are instructed as to the importance of joining and empathically listening to their clients, most therapists are relieved, feeling "I can do that!"

Finally, beginning therapists need to recognize that their early experiences in seeing clients often involve a steep learning curve, like any other new job. You will be less anxious doing an intake with a family if you have one or two intakes "under your belt." It takes time, however, to gain enough experience so that many situations become familiar.

Many beginning therapists wonder at what point they will stop struggling with issues of confidence. Experienced clinicians indicated that after 5 to 7 years (or about 5,000 to 7,000 hours) of clinical experience, they had encountered most clinical issues or problems several times. As a result, they felt very secure or confident in their abilities as therapists.

Fortunately, therapists don't need to complete 5,000 to 7,000 hours of work to see a notable improvement in their confidence. The intense feelings of anxiety and being overwhelmed that are common in the beginning generally subside after a month or so of seeing clients. Beginning therapists also become less fearful that they will do something to harm their clients, although they continue to struggle with feelings of being ineffective or unhelpful.

Obtaining 500 to 700 hours appears to be another significant turning point in the growth of therapist confidence. At this level of experience, beginning therapists generally report greater confidence in conceptualizing cases. They often report knowing what needs to be changed, but are unsure of how to intervene to bring that change about.

Most therapists will have confidence in their overall abilities by the time they have had 1,000 to 1,500 hours of clinical experience. At this point, they are better at conceptualizing cases and have also developed a repertoire of effective interventions. Of course, therapists can still experience periodic doubts about their abilities, particularly when struggling with difficult cases or issues. Issues of confidence may also reemerge if therapists start working with new and unfamiliar populations. However, most therapists at this stage are not plagued by doubts about their clinical ability.

STAGES OF THERAPIST DEVELOPMENT

McCollum (1990) notes that therapists trained in individual therapy generally go through three stages of development when learning to do family therapy. In the first stage, they focus on acquiring the skills necessary to work with families. In the second stage, they learn to apply systemic theory to their clinical work, and in the third, "self of the therapist" stage, they focus on more personal issues in relationship to their clinical work, such as exploring how their family of origin experiences affect their work with families.

Although McCollum's observations were based on teaching experienced therapists to do family therapy, these stages also apply to individuals learning family therapy without prior clinical experience. In essence, the initial skills stage is characterized by the therapist trying to figure out what to do with clients. This focus then shifts in the theory stage to how to think. In the final stage, the therapist focuses on the use of self in being with a family.

Although each stage has a particular emphasis, all three may overlap from time to time. While developmental stages are differentiated by time and experience, other factors can bring any or all of their foci to the forefront—particular client families and clinical issues, the emphasis of a certain supervisor or training program, and the abiding interests of the therapist, among others.

Stage One: Learning Essential Skills

Before therapists start their clinical work, they often experience a mixture of feelings. Most report an excitement at finally beginning to "do" therapy, and some even express impatience to see clients. They are eager to apply what they have learned in their classes by working with people in therapy. However, the predominant emotion that most therapists report before seeing their first client is significant anxiety.

It is natural for therapists to have these worries before they see their first client and even after they begin to work. Beginning therapists report feeling overwhelmed by the experience. Many report going home after seeing clients and crying, while others report that the stress results in headaches, difficulty sleeping, stomachaches, or changes in appetite.

This early stage is a time for beginners to learn and practice basic skills. Learning to relax and be present in the therapy room with clients is a good place to start. A solid assessment and effective treatment hinge on the therapist's ability to listen and attend to the client's story, and to show the client that he or she is understood. Beginners can learn to replace their anxiety about "doing something" with relaxed curiosity and empathy. This approach leads to useful questions and inquiries, which is where therapy begins.

Stage Two: Learning to Conceptualize Cases

Beginning therapists soon recognize that the therapeutic relationship is a necessary but not always sufficient ingredient for change. They no longer are content simply to be with their clients; they realize that some clients need concrete ideas or suggestions for change. At the same time, therapists also become aware that to be effective, interventions must be rooted in a clear understanding of family dynamics. As a result, therapists soon move into a second stage, where emphasis is placed on conceptualizing what is happening in their cases.

Learning to conceptualize cases can be difficult and frustrating. In this stage, therapists frequently struggle with issues such as the following:

"How do I know what is the most important information to attend
to in a case?"

"My clients keep coming in with a different problem each week.
How do I figure out what to focus on?"

"I know I should have a theory for this case, but I'm not sure what
theory would 'work' here."

"I thought I knew what we should be working on last week, but
now I'm confused again."

"I know I should be focusing on the process, but I feel like I'm
stuck in the content."

Typically, beginning therapists are able to develop good insights
and hypotheses, but will have difficulty connecting these pieces
together into a coherent picture or treatment plan. Gradually, there
will be moments of clarity when the pieces fit together. With the passage of time, these moments begin to last longer than the periods of
haze and confusion.

Early in the second stage, many therapists find it helpful to adopt
a particular theoretical orientation for conceptualizing cases (McCollum, 1990). As they gain intensive experience with one theoretical
framework, they begin to recognize its limitations and may try others.
As therapists explore different theories, they eventually develop their
own framework, integrating the best parts of the different orientations
that they have adopted.

Stage Three: The Therapist-as-Self

As therapists become more skilled at and comfortable with conceptualizing cases, they shift more of their focus to looking at themselves in
therapy. There is a growing recognition that the self of the therapist
can greatly influence therapy, and beginning family therapists gradually become more interested in identifying their unique contributions
to the therapeutic encounter.

During this stage, therapists will often explore how the therapist-
as-self is both an asset and liability in therapy. Many of our personal
experiences can become catalysts for new ideas and understanding
in therapeutic work. For example, a therapist who has been able to
successfully develop an adult-to-adult relationship with his or her parents may use that personal experience in working with clients who
are struggling with issues of differentiation. Specific life experiences—
trauma, parenthood, separation, illness—may all come into play in a
way that benefits therapeutic work.

However, therapists' unresolved issues or "growth areas" can become impediments in therapy. Therefore, some therapists choose to explore their personal issues more closely at this stage, often by seeking therapy for themselves. The growth and insight derived from working on these issues can provide the perspective necessary to make constructive use of life experiences in therapy.

OBSESSING ABOUT CLINICAL WORK

Many beginning therapists report that they cannot stop thinking about therapy or their clients. In fact, thinking about clients seems to fill every waking moment and even many nonwaking moments. It is not unusual for beginning therapists to report having dreams about their clients or about doing therapy.

Learning to do anything new, particularly something as challenging as therapy, can easily consume much of one's time, attention, and energy. Furthermore, most people who choose therapy as a profession have a deep compassion and concern for people. It is often difficult not to think about clients, particularly when they are in considerable pain or distress.

Thinking (or even obsessing) about clients is something that tends to subside with time and experience. Most experienced therapists report thinking very little about their clients outside the therapy hour. One reason for this change is that the therapist gradually gains a greater sense of clinical mastery by virtue of experience. In addition, therapists learn to balance objectivity and emotional involvement with clients. In a sense, therapists learn how to construct an emotional boundary (Skovholt & Rønnestad, 2003). If the boundary becomes too diffuse, the therapist may be overwhelmed and inducted into the family system. If it is too rigid, he or she may lack the empathy necessary to adequately understand the issues and join with the family. The former problem is characteristic of beginning therapists, who, with time, learn to better regulate this boundary.

DEALING WITH BURNOUT

At first glance, one would not anticipate that someone who is just beginning a career as a family therapist would experience feelings of burnout. Yet many beginning therapists experience some degree of burnout during their clinical training. It is not uncommon for individuals struggling with burnout even to question whether they want to continue their careers as therapists. The potential for burnout among beginning therapists exists because of several factors.

First, learning to do therapy can be demanding. Worrying about one's competence as a beginning therapist can take its toll over time, perhaps diminishing some of the enjoyment of doing therapy. Beginning therapists may also overextend themselves or worry excessively about their clients until they learn to better manage their emotional boundaries.

Second, therapists have other stressors outside of their clinical work. For example, you may have other classes, comprehensive exams, or a master's or doctoral thesis to complete as part of your training program. You may need to work to pay for school or living expenses, or may have a family or partner who needs your time and energy. You may experience considerable stress from trying to successfully meet all these commitments.

Third, the courses or clinical work may raise personal issues for you as you learn to do therapy. Insights gained from clinical training inevitably lead student therapists to reexamine their own lives and families. Although this process can become the catalyst for significant personal growth, it can also place one more additional demand on the beginning therapist.

In order to avoid burnout, practicing good self-care is essential (Norcross & Guy, 2007). For example, you need to build in time for "recharging your batteries." Individuals who are faced with extreme time demands often put off taking personal time to do this. Taking time for yourself seems counterintuitive when faced with an overwhelming number of tasks to accomplish, but the time lost is often made up by being able to work with renewed energy and efficiency. Ironically, many therapists are willing to give this advice to their clients but have difficulty following it themselves.

Being willing to set limits is another important tool to avoid burnout. Beginning therapists often report setting their client schedule based largely on the convenience of their clients. In some cases, beginning therapists come in 5 days a week even though their caseload requires only 3 or 4 days. As therapists gain experience, they often will become more willing to set some limits on their availability, giving them some protected time for themselves.

You also need a strong social support network. Many of us owe our families a great deal of credit for the emotional and financial support they provided during our training. However, you also need support and understanding that others who are not therapists cannot always provide. Both experienced and inexperienced therapists need colleagues with whom they can share clinical experiences to avoid burnout.

THE BIG PICTURE

This chapter has identified some of the common challenges that beginning therapists encounter early in their careers. While dealing with these challenges, it's important to keep the "big picture" in mind and recall the benefits of being a therapist. Learning to do therapy can be a strong catalyst for personal growth. What one learns about helping other families can be applied to one's own life and family, making it more enriching. As a therapist, you will be privileged to witness deeply moving moments of courage and compassion on the part of your clients. It is rewarding to see individuals create more fulfilling lives, knowing that we contributed in part to this growth or change. Often the clients whom we struggle the most to help are the ones who give us the greatest sense of fulfillment when they actually do succeed in changing. As you move through the rough spots, it can be helpful to keep the following "reminders" at hand:

1. *Becoming a therapist takes time.* This is an opportunity for you to be a learner; you are not expected to be an expert. Becoming an effective therapist takes several years of training.
2. *Make sure you take care of yourself.* Use constructive means for stress reduction. Develop resources for support from other students, peers, and colleagues.
3. *Self-doubts are normal.* Be patient with yourself, focus on the positive, and pay attention to the developmental tasks of becoming a therapist.
4. *Use the skills that brought you to the field.* While you are learning lots of new theory and material, continue to pay attention to your intuition, your desire to work with others, and your natural abilities.

CONCLUSION

Building confidence and competence in one's clinical work is part of the larger process of learning to do good therapy. The greatest task for a beginning family therapist lies in developing a clear understanding of clinical issues and an ability to apply therapeutic skills, to which we devote the remainder of this book.

Chapters 2–6 follow the usual time sequence of therapy—from initial contact with clients, to comprehensive assessment, to treatment planning and intervention. Mental health skills needed by all therapists are intertwined with family therapy knowledge. Our goal here is to provide beginning therapists with the tools for thinking about clinical issues, rather than merely applying an approach propounded by their instructors.

Chapters 7–9 deal with specific clinical situations based on presenting problems and the nature of client families. We examine major issues and approaches for working with children and adolescents, couples, and families that are struggling with serious mental illness.

Chapter 10 highlights some common obstacles all therapists encounter, and provides concrete ideas on how to get unstuck when treatment is not progressing. Chapter 11 focuses on an often overlooked part of therapy—termination. In Chapter 12, we conclude the book by looking at emerging issues within family therapy. We believe that beginning therapists should pay attention to these emerging themes so they can continue to grow along with the field in providing clients the best possible care.

CHAPTER 2

Before the Initial Interview

M rs. Escutia's voice quivers nervously over the phone line at a community counseling clinic. "I must speak to a counselor ... please!" she exclaims. "My grandson is in trouble, he needs help. I don't know what to do anymore. I'm afraid he could ... " The clinic intake worker jots down a few notes and quickly calls up one of the clinic's family therapy interns. "I've got a woman on the phone whose grandson just put his fist through a wall," the intake worker says. "Can you take her?" For a brief moment, the new client and the new intern share a silent space filled with questions and anxieties. The first contact is about to take place, and it can easily make or break a future collaboration where healing work can be done.

DEALING WITH FAMILIES' EXPECTATIONS AND ANXIETIES ABOUT THERAPY

The moment captured in the preceding case material provides a glimpse of one of the most critical points in the therapeutic experience—the period before therapy ever begins. It is during this fragile period that prospective clients decide if they want to risk going to therapy. While clients with previous positive therapy experiences may reinitiate treatment with a hopeful attitude, others are ambivalent in their hopes, expectations, and fears about beginning therapy.

Consider Mrs. Escutia. In her family, problems have traditionally been handled by husbands and wives, aunts and uncles, grandparents, longtime friends, and others who are close to the family hearth. Her anxiety about calling in "professional" help is matched only by her concern for her grandson, whose violent temper has pushed the entire family past its limits. With no previous experience in therapy, she wonders what a stranger in this clinic could possibly do to help—after all, everything has been tried! Will this counselor believe her? How should she present this terrible dilemma? Will anyone out there really care? Does seeking help mean she has failed?

It is not uncommon for families to be at their wit's end when they finally decide to seek treatment or are referred and call for an appointment. Chances are they're worn out, fed up, and feeling hopeless. Further, individual family members may differ remarkably in their attitudes, expectations, and motivations regarding a try at therapy. They may have both overt and covert reasons for coming to therapy, and rarely are the family members' reasons the same. Much of this information may not be uncovered until the first interview or even beyond, but it is a good idea to keep the following questions in mind right from the first contact:

"What are the clients' expectations about therapy?"
"What are their anxieties about coming to therapy?"
"What motivates them to come to therapy, and who is the referral source?"
"Why do they want to come to therapy now?"

If the therapist isn't aware of the often hidden issues related to clients' motivation, expectations, and anxieties, he or she may inadvertently respond in a manner that causes clients to decide that therapy is not worth the risk, or, conversely, that leads to accepting clients who might be better served elsewhere. For example, beginning therapists may find themselves drawn into legal cases that involve divorce, custody, adoption, or numerous other types of litigation. Family therapists are seldom trained in the specifics of mediation or custody evaluation, and, for most of us, it is best to decline doing therapy in such situations.

Even in cases where therapy is clearly indicated and doesn't involve potential legal tangles, family members' reasons for starting treatment and levels of motivation are important to assess. In individual work, these issues may be less salient because rarely do individuals come to therapy without wanting to be there. Conjoint treatment presents a different picture. For example, in couple therapy there is often one person who is more motivated to come to therapy or at least views therapy as an effective method for dealing with relationship problems. The partner may be resistant to treatment, have other preferred solutions for addressing marital issues, or be willing to come to therapy only if it is framed as a way to "help my partner" or "save the marriage."

With families, reasons and motivations for therapy vary further. Perhaps one powerful family member is coercing others to attend. Perhaps the safety of a "neutral" therapist and a scheduled weekly hour is necessary for a family to talk together about personal and significant issues. In addition, referral sources and previous treatment are absolutely crucial to consider when gauging family members' diverse responses to seeing a therapist. Court-ordered treatment may indicate a potentially resistant or reluctant client, though this is by no means the rule. Referrals by school counselors, ministers, physicians, or family friends will likely influence how families first approach treatment. For example, family members may not agree with a school counselor's view of "the problem" and as a result have little investment in seeking therapy. On the other hand, such a referral from a perceived professional may be just the validation the family needs to actively seek help. Similarly, the nature of previous contacts with other agencies or individuals may predispose a family to have enormous expectations for therapy, or none at all. Since these rarely articulated expectations and anxieties will alter how a therapist approaches treatment with a new family, it is essential to get a feel for them from the outset.

Clients like Mrs. Escutia will have as many questions swirling about as the therapist does when the first contact is made. Topping the list may be concerns about the therapist's ability to truly understand and care, and questions about whether he or she can actually help. Clients may find answers to these questions in how quickly their phone calls are returned or in their sense that the listener understands a brief explanation of the problem. The therapist's (or agency's) flexibility in responding to individual needs communicates answers to these questions. The degree of focus on charges and payments versus listening to the client may communicate that the client is not a priority—money is. If the client decides, via these early perceptions, that the therapist doesn't care or can't help, the initial session may never happen. On the other hand, an initial call that relays empathy and confidence can begin to create the foundation upon which a successful therapy can be built.

SUGGESTIONS FOR INITIAL CONTACT WITH THE CLIENT

Keeping in mind the myriad expectations, anxieties, and questions of potential clients, therapists can be guided through the first-time telephone conversation by using a number of pragmatic suggestions for handling initial contacts:

1. *Listen and reflect to the client what you hear.* Simply by listening and briefly reflecting what is said, you can help the prospective client feel he or she has been heard. Effective listening can be done in 5 minutes, and the client can hang up with a new sense of hope about resolving the problem.

2. *Assess if this is a crisis situation.* The initial phone call may indicate a need for immediate crisis intervention, hospitalization, removal of family members from the home, or involvement of other agencies such as police or child protective services. Therapists should be knowledgeable about the clinic's or agency's protocol for handling crises, and about community or state laws that may apply (e.g., child abuse reporting laws).

3. *Consider scope-of-practice issues.* Do you have the knowledge and experience to diagnose and treat the presenting problem? Some agencies carefully screen the clients that beginning therapists treat. For example, a problem that is primarily biomedical, one that involves suicide risk or serious drug or alcohol use, or a purely individualized problem (such as a phobia) may not be within the scope of practice for a marriage and family therapist. You can begin clarifying your strengths and limits immediately.

4. *Respond as promptly as possible.* Return phone calls, set up the initial session, and complete an assessment as quickly as you can. These behaviors indicate that you take the client's concerns seriously and are competent to respond to his or her needs. You create a sense of credibility and assure the client that you can help early on.

5. *Consider why this particular family member made the initial contact, and keep in mind that a sense of rapport with each individual in the family is important.* Therapists often make several mistakes around this issue. It is easy to be drawn to the most "psychologically minded" or powerful client and inadvertently ignore those who are likely part of the problem as well as part of the solution. Before the first session, the family member who made the phone call is in essence the family spokesperson. However, the therapist may want contact with other family members before the first session. The goal of additional phone contacts is to make sure every family member feels welcome and knows that his or her feelings and ideas matter to the therapist.

6. *Address the "business" of therapy as quickly and efficiently as possible while not detracting from the client's need to be heard.* Basic explanations about fees and payment, how to make appointments, and policies about keeping and canceling appointments are important. Transportation issues are relevant for many families, too. Do the clients have a car, or someone who can drive them to appointments? Must they navigate and pay for public transportation? Do they have directions to the clinic? What about family work and school schedules? Do they

have childcare, if this is needed? Addressing such concerns up front can assist the therapist and family in avoiding no-shows and cancellations due to logistical problems that were never worked out. Issues such as informed consent and confidentiality may be dealt with on the telephone, or more frequently through mailed information or forms provided at the clinic just before the first session. (Chapter 3 addresses these issues in detail.) Regardless of how this information is communicated, it is important to ensure that clients are clearly informed about what is expected of them and what they can expect from therapy.

7. *Limit the first contact by sticking to basic, relevant information and issues.* This is not the time to offer interventions, advice, or suggestions. Be prepared to direct the telephone interview. Prospective clients may be interested in lengthy venting of problems, in getting detailed information about your qualifications, methods, and philosophy, or in obtaining an immediate diagnosis, or they may have other concerns that, while valid, are best saved for a first meeting. You want to make the client feel understood but also focus on the opportunity to explore the problems in more depth in your initial meeting. Typically, clients' anxiety will be significantly reduced once they know they have an appointment and a place to discuss their concerns.

WHAT INFORMATION SHOULD BE OBTAINED?

Most agencies and therapists have an intake form that gathers basic information about the client during the initial contact. This information may be obtained by an intake receptionist or a therapist over the phone. Other possibilities include mailing the form to the client before the first session or having the client complete the form in the waiting room before the first session. Even though initial telephone contacts are time-limited and may not be as comprehensive as formal intake questionnaires, the call can still begin the processes of evaluation and joining by focusing on the following questions:

1. What is the problem and how does the client present it? Is this a crisis, a severe or moderate problem, a discrete situation, a chronic difficulty?
2. How has the family responded to the situation? How have they managed so far?
3. Has there been previous therapy?
4. Why is the family seeking treatment now?
5. What additional factors are influencing the situation (e.g., nature and frequency of various stressors—whether they are vocational, personal, physical, or otherwise)?

Figure 2.1 provides a sample intake form that reflects the information deemed most important by marriage and family therapists. The emphasis on specific information varies, depending on the training of the mental health professional. For example, most psychiatric intake forms focus on individual symptoms instead of relationships, whereas a child psychologist may include questions about a child's prenatal history and delivery. Regardless of the therapist's orientation, all intake forms should include a place for the client's brief description of the problem (in the client's own words), notes about previous treatments, and inquiries about current medications and medical problems. Whether this information is obtained during an initial phone contact or at the first session, it is crucial data that helps direct assessment and treatment.

WHO SHOULD COME TO THERAPY?

During the initial phone contact, the therapist needs to indicate that involvement of the family is critical. While most therapists are flexible enough not to insist that everyone involved be present at every session, an early message that therapy is usually a family affair lays the groundwork for involvement by members who may be perceived as peripheral to the problem. When the presenting problem clearly involves a relationship (sibling fights or parent–child standoffs), it is a useful general rule to get all the people in the relationship to come to therapy.

Beyond this basic principle, the following guidelines can help you determine, early on, the best possible format for new clients:

1. Ask the family who they want to come to therapy, and why.
2. Try and identify who in the family is impacted by the current problems. Ask if they might want to come to a session.
3. Consider generational boundaries. Is it appropriate to have all age groups in therapy?
4. Even if the problem is primarily an individual one, would other family members' presence facilitate treatment or feel supportive to the individual?
5. Would other family members hinder the therapy and be potentially damaging?
6. What motivation and capacity does the family have to participate in a family format?
7. Be open to changing who comes for each session depending on the problem, but try to establish a relationship with all members.

Name: Telephone: Date of Birth: Place of Birth: Age:

Address: Marital Status: Religion: Race: Gender:

Place of Employment: Length of Employment:

Last Place of Employment: Length of Employment:

Address: Supervisor:

Telephone: Hours Worked: Salary:

Education Completed: Where:

Name(s) of Child/   Date of Birth: Age: School Attended:
Children:

Have you (or your spouse) ever been involved in therapy or any other type of counseling program? ☐ Yes ☐ No

If yes, when? _____ Where? _____

Reasons: _____

Reasons for considering counseling at this time: _____

Have you been referred to this agency before? ☐ Yes ☐ No If yes, by whom? _____

Reasons for the referral: _____

Are you in treatment with another counselor at this time? ☐ Yes ☐ No If yes, with whom? _____

When? _____ How long? _____

Have you ever been hospitalized for any mental health problems? ☐ Yes ☐ No
If yes, when? _____

Where? _____ By whom? _____

Have you ever been, or are you now being, treated for any type of chemical dependency or abuse? ☐ Yes ☐ No

If yes, when? _____ Where? _____

(cont.)

FIGURE 2.1. **Sample intake form.**

By whom? _____ Length of treatment? _____

Are you at the present time using any type of chemical substance? ☐ Yes ☐ No
If yes, please indicate what you are using (drugs and/or alcohol): _____

How frequently do you use these substances? _____

Are you presently under a physician's care for physical problems? ☐ Yes ☐ No
If yes, please list medication: _____

Name of family physician: _____ Telephone: _____

Address: _____

Have you ever been arrested and/or committed a crime? ☐ Yes ☐ No

If yes, when? _____ For what? _____

Outcome of situation: _____

What problems are you presently experiencing? _____
_____

What do you expect from therapy? _____
_____

Please list everyone in your family with whom you presently live:

_____ _____
_____ _____
_____ _____
_____ _____

Identify the primary problem(s) you are now experiencing: _____
_____

If need be, would other relatives be willing to come in to therapy sessions? ☐ Yes ☐ No

If no, please indicate reason: _____

Person to contact in case of emergency: _____ Telephone: _____

Address: _____

_____   _____
Signature   Date

TO ALL CLIENTS:

If any concerns arise about your treatment, please discuss them with your therapist.

Intake comments:

Preliminary treatment plans:

FIGURE 2.1. *(cont.)*

Clients naturally have an opinion about who should come to therapy, and the reasons underlying such views should be considered and addressed. For example, sometimes a spouse will request individual therapy "because I'm the one causing the problems in the marriage." The therapist can point out that a relationship problem is involved and can recommend that both partners attend. Similarly, family members may consider the "identified patient" to be the only one who needs to come to therapy. Clearly, a direct relationship exists between treatment goals and who attends therapy. Therapy goals may be limited or broadened depending on the willingness of different family members to participate in therapy. As long as the relationship between participation and goals is clarified for the family when the terms of therapy are being established, there need not be any hard-and-fast rules about who comes to each session.

In a survey of marriage and family therapists, Doherty and Simmons (1996) reported that family therapists are most likely to see, in rank order, individuals, then couples, then families. Northey (2002) confirmed those findings in another survey of American Association for Marriage and Family Therapy (AAMFT) clinical members, finding "clients being seen individually 54% of the time and in couple and family sessions between 35% and 42% of the time respectively" (p. 493). Marital and family problems were seen as the most common presenting problems. It seems that the public is beginning to conceptualize problems as being relational rather than primarily individual. Radio and television talk shows, as well as many popular magazines and movies, have emphasized the relational nature of mental health problems, and there appears to be a greater willingness to look at the stresses of normal relationships as well as dysfunctional ones. Therapists may need to educate new clients about the benefits of conjoint treatment by emphasizing the power of relationships in influencing how people feel, think, and act. The role that social and cultural factors play in creating relationship difficulties may also need to be discussed. While there are many times when individual therapy is appropriate, family therapists generally focus their treatment on relationships by having more than one person present. When a marriage and family therapist is working individually, he or she is likely to take a systemic view of the case, which means that the focus of the therapy will include looking at the main players and social systems involved in the client's life.

INITIAL HYPOTHESIZING

After the initial contact, most therapists find themselves with enough basic information to begin forming a few hypotheses, which provide them with areas to pursue further in the first interview. Questions should be designed to elicit data that will either support or invalidate the hypotheses.

In order to begin the process of clinical thinking, the therapist needs to pay close attention to what is known and how that information might be useful. Too often we look quickly for underlying meanings of events before we have a working understanding of the presenting problem. It can be helpful to first summarize what information is available and then pick out the key issues. What is the client telling you that he or she thinks is important? Initially, the process of asking key questions will prove far more fruitful than making interpretations of the client's motives or behavior.

-The process of developing hypotheses is an opportunity for creative thinking. Our guesses and speculations are based upon our previous experiences with similar cases, our knowledge about individual or family development, and our clinical hunches or intuitions. At this stage of the process, we are not looking for answers, but finding questions. Hypotheses relate to what may be happening or what events could have occurred. The therapist's position is not to presume to know, but to form some hunches and then ask. The following example of a clinical situation shows how developing some hypotheses proves useful in beginning a clinical assessment.

A 9-year-old girl who has never really liked school suddenly refuses to go at all. She has become withdrawn and sullen. When asked why she doesn't want to go to school, she simply cries and refuses to answer. In order to develop some hypotheses about this case, it is first useful to note and summarize the key issues. The presenting problem is the child's refusal to go to school. Her response to being asked about the problem is to cry and withdraw. A key word in the vignette is "suddenly." That this change was abrupt is critical information for developing our hypotheses. A sudden change in her attitude and behavior can lead to speculation that something uncomfortable and possibly traumatic has occurred. Her difficulty in responding to questions about her behavior would add fuel to the notion that something frightening has happened and that she is withdrawing from it. These are some of the hypotheses for the clinician to explore. Others might be the following:

1. The girl is being intimidated by someone at school.
2. An abrupt change has occurred at home and she wants to be there.
3. She is developing a school phobia.

4. She is depressed and her school difficulties are symptomatic of her depression.
5. She has a physical problem that she is afraid to talk about.

These hypotheses provide the therapist with possible explanations for the changes in her behavior. They provide direction for further inquiry, but are not intended to be a complete list. Hypotheses help narrow our focus and rule out possibilities. Once a few hypotheses have been developed, the therapist can begin to think about what additional information might prove helpful. Being curious about a client can be a useful, nonevaluative position for the therapist's inquiry. Similarly, in consultations, supervisors and colleagues can suggest directions to take and questions to pursue. In addition, even preliminary information may suggest the need for referrals for physical examinations, psychological testing, or developmental evaluation.

CONCLUSION

Therapy begins with the first contact, before the clients ever meet with their therapist. The clients begin to form impressions about therapy and the therapist. In addition, the therapist can start gathering information for initial hypothesizing. We recently talked to a client new to therapy. She said that the warmth in the voice of the intake administrator and the warmth of the waiting room immediately made her feel safe. She was ready to begin therapy. A student therapist told us that her new clients started arguing about their son as she walked them from the waiting room to her office. She wondered what that meant. We recommend that you consider any contact the clients have with you or your agency starting with the first phone call. Handling early interactions well can set a positive tone for the rest of the therapy.

CHAPTER 3

The Initial Interview

It is 5 minutes to the hour when she looks anxiously at the clock, just before the first session. For what feels like the thousandth time, she mentally rehearses exactly what she wants to say at the beginning of the session. She is worried that she will forget something important because of nervousness. She desperately wants to make a good impression. It is now 2 minutes to the hour—if only the butterflies in her stomach would disappear, she might feel ready. She looks at the door, and wishes for a brief second that she could leave. She takes a deep breath as the door to the therapy office opens ...

Did you imagine this to be the client or the therapist waiting for the first session to begin? Either could be true. For therapists and clients alike, beginning therapy can elicit feelings of fear, excitement, and nervous anticipation. Each client will take you on a different journey. This chapter covers the basic issues that must be addressed in the initial interview to ensure that your journey gets off to a good start.

STAGES OF THE INITIAL INTERVIEW

Many beginning therapists find it helpful to think of the initial interview in stages. In the first stage, the therapist welcomes the client, couple, or family to therapy. The goal of this stage is to do introductions and put the clients at ease. Administrative issues are addressed in the second stage. The purpose of this stage is to ensure clients have a clear understanding of the therapy process, including confidentiality, videotaping, and fees. After covering administrative issues, the therapist can transition to the goal-setting phase. Here the therapist learns what the clients hope to accomplish through therapy. Once a good understanding of client goals and expectations for therapy has been reached, the therapist can begin the assessment phase, which typically extends beyond the first interview.

The length of time devoted to each phase can vary greatly from client to client. Often the first two stages of the initial interview, welcoming the client and handling administrative issues, can be accomplished within the first 10–15 minutes. In some cases, however, clients may have a lot of questions about the therapy process, which may extend the second stage. The length of the goal-setting stage can depend upon several factors. Some clients will be able to succinctly state their concerns, while others will go off on tangents or long stories about the presenting issues. The time devoted to goal setting will also depend upon the number of clients being seen. Soliciting everyone's perspective on goals within a family will generally take longer than working with an individual. In most cases the therapist will be able to devote some time to assessment in the initial interview. However, with some clients, simply being able to establish goals for therapy is a realistic expectation.

You will need to accomplish several important tasks to make the initial interview successful. Some tasks, like goal setting, will fit nicely within a particular stage. Other tasks, however, may not fit easily within a particular stage, or may require attention across multiple stages of the initial interview. For example, you should be working on building your relationship with your clients, at each stage of the initial interview. Important assessment information may also come out at any point in the first session, even before the therapist has begun a more formal assessment phase.

DEVELOPING A CONNECTION: HOW TO JOIN WITH CLIENTS

The most crucial task in the first session is for you to successfully join with your clients. *Joining* means that clients feel a sense of connectedness with you, which usually arises when they feel that you understand, respect, and care about them. The importance of joining cannot be overstated: It is the foundation for future work. Failure to successfully join with your clients will hamper all of your efforts, from assessment to treatment. For example, clients will be reluctant to share sensitive information if you have not established a safe and secure relationship with them. Likewise, clients may become highly resistant to or defensive toward suggestions if you have not created a strong therapeutic relationship with them. Ultimately, failure to join with clients will likely lead to premature termination of therapy.

Joining is a process that should be carefully attended to throughout the entire initial interview. It begins in the first moments of therapy, as clients are welcomed into your office. You should attempt to put your clients at ease, since they are most likely anxious about coming to therapy. You might engage in some brief social talk with them to break the ice before discussing problems. You might ask them, for example, what kind of work they do or what they like to do for fun. Besides making your clients feel comfortable talking with you, this approach demonstrates your personal interest in them. You might also share some information about yourself so that the clients can get to know you. Ideally, you will be able to identify something you have in common with your clients that will help develop a sense of connection.

Joining can also take place at other points throughout the initial interview. For example, joining can occur when you respectfully listen to and address questions your clients have about confidentiality, fees, and other issues. Likewise, giving each of your clients an opportunity to tell his or her story can facilitate joining by allowing each person to feel heard and understood. Reflective listening, maintaining direct eye contact, or leaning forward can also reinforce to your clients that you are interested in and concerned about what they are saying. Concluding the initial interview with a positive message for your clients can be another way to strengthen your connection. For example, a husband who resists coming to therapy can be complimented for caring enough about his relationship to come despite his strong reservations about therapy.

Although skills to facilitate joining can be learned, it is important to recognize that developing a relationship with another person cannot be reduced to a recipe or set of techniques. In fact, the greatest asset any therapist brings to the process is him- or herself. Your personality, attitudes, life experiences, and mannerisms become a part of and help create the relationship.

Although the therapist's personality is usually an asset to promoting joining, there are times when therapist characteristics can create a barrier to developing a connection. Therapists who have prejudices or negative preconceptions about people based on race, ethnicity, sexual orientation, socioeconomic status, or religious orientation will likely have difficulty establishing a connection with clients who have these characteristics. Likewise, therapists may have a difficult time joining with a client who reminds them of someone with whom they had a painful relationship (perhaps a parent or spouse). Therefore, you should be vigilant in assuring that personal issues or prejudices do not interfere with your developing a relationship with your clients.

HANDLING ADMINISTRATIVE ISSUES

One of the early tasks in an initial interview is to address administrative issues so clients understand the therapy process. Although these matters are typically called administrative issues, it is important to recognize that therapeutic issues are frequently played out through them. One client who was adamant about not being videotaped was discovered through further assessment to have a high level of distrust toward people, which became a key area of focus in therapy. Therefore, the therapist who is attuned to the process and not just the content when handling administrative issues may discover important opportunities for assessment or even intervention.

Confidentiality and Release of Information

You should always address the issue of confidentiality with your clients. They need to be informed not only of the confidential nature of therapy, but also of the possible circumstances in which confidentiality will be broken (e.g., threat of harm to self or others, child abuse, elder/dependent abuse). As discussed in Chapter 2, information on confidentiality may be included on a client information form that can be mailed to clients prior to the first session, or read by them in the office before the first session.

Therapists working with couples and families must also consider how confidentiality among family members will be handled. Some therapists, for example, will conduct individual sessions as part of a couple's treatment. Likewise, a therapist may meet individually with a child or adolescent in addition to family treatment. The therapist must address the extent to which information obtained during these individual sessions will be kept confidential or shared with other family members. Some therapists insist on a "no-secrets policy" between family members, while others allow information learned in individual sessions to remain confidential. Regardless of one's position, it is best to offer clear written and verbal guidelines as to the bounds of confidentiality at the beginning of therapy.

You will frequently want to consult with other individuals or institutions connected with particular cases, such as previous therapists, psychiatrists or physicians, school officials or teachers, lawyers, courts, and parole officers. In these cases, you will need to have clients sign a release of information form, such as the one depicted in Figure 3.1, to permit communication between you and the other parties. The signatures of all participants in therapy are required for the release of information. For example, you should obtain *both* the husband's and wife's

To: _____
　　　　　　(practitioner, hospital, etc.)

I have been informed that under _____ (state) law, communications between a client and his or her therapist are privileged and may not be disclosed by the therapist unless the client consents. I also have been informed that client records maintained by a therapist may not be disclosed to third parties except with the client's consent or through legal process.

I authorize _____ (name of therapist) to share information and/ or records about my therapy to _____ (name of person or entity to whom the disclosure will be made).

I am permitting authorized disclosure of information about my therapy for the following purposes:

_____

_____

_____

I am permitting authorized disclosure of the following types of information (choose one):

___ All information or records related to my therapy

___ Only the following information (please specify)

_____

_____

_____

This authorization shall remain in effect until _____ (date). I understand that any cancellation or modification of this authorization must be in writing.

_____
Date

_____
Client name (printed)

_____
Client signature

_____　　　_____
Witnessed by　　　　　　　　　　　　　　　　　Date

FIGURE 3.1. Authorization for release of information.

signatures if both have been participants in the course of therapy. If others contact you about your clients, you should not even acknowledge that they are in therapy unless you have obtained the appropriate release of information.

Therapeutic issues may arise when discussing confidentiality with clients. For example, if a husband or wife in couple therapy inquires if the court can obtain therapy records, you might suspect that one of the partners is seriously thinking of divorce.

Videotaping and Observation

Beginning family therapists are frequently instructed to videotape all or some of their sessions for supervision purposes. The vast majority of clients agree to be videotaped if they are approached properly about it. Explain why the videotaping is beneficial to both therapist and client, and address issues of confidentiality regarding videotaping. You can tell your clients that you regularly consult with other therapists, and that videotaping allows them to witness firsthand what happened in therapy. You can then explain that consulting with therapists in this manner is helpful to both you and your clients since "two heads are better than one." You can add that videotaping allows you to review what happened in previous sessions and perhaps have a new insight, much like people notice something new when watching a movie for the second time. Finally, point out that videotaping the session allows the couple or family to see how they interact when they watch a replay.

You should inform the client of who will view the videotape, emphasizing that videotapes are considered confidential information. Indicate as well what will happen to the tapes after the completion of therapy, assuring clients that videotapes are not kept permanently, but are regularly erased or recorded over. Clients should be asked to sign a form giving their consent for videotaping. The form should outline the purpose of the videotaping, who will view the videotape, and what will happen to the tapes after therapy is completed.

In a small number of cases, clients may be reluctant to be videotaped. You should carefully explore their reasons with them. In many cases, clients may simply be hesitant due to self-consciousness. Most of these clients will be agreeable to being videotaped if assured that their reaction is a common one and that people generally forget about the camera in a short time. You should pay careful attention to clients who are insistent about not being videotaped since they are the exception rather than the rule. These clients often have sensitive information that they wish to protect or keep secret. For example, one client who refused to be videotaped disclosed indirectly that he had engaged in illegal activities. In some cases, clients will agree to be videotaped if you will turn off the video camera when they indicate that they are ready to disclose particularly sensitive information. If a client is not open to videotaping under any circumstances, you should respect this decision in order to avoid damaging the therapeutic relationship and possibly precipitating a premature termination of therapy. Clients may agree to be videotaped once they have established greater trust in you or the therapeutic process.

If therapy will include live supervision or the use of observing/reflecting teams, discuss this with your clients. Most of them will agree to this format if they are told why the supervision or team benefits both therapist and client. It is often helpful to allow clients, at their request, to meet supervisors or team members who observe the sessions from behind the one-way mirror.

Fees

Determining the client's fee can be an uncomfortable process. It is difficult to assign a monetary value to therapy, and therapists often feel uneasy about charging fees while acting in a helping role. Therapist anxiety about fees can easily be transferred to clients and can create conflict and stress in therapy. Comfort in handling fees will increase with therapeutic experience and confidence in your ability to provide a worthwhile service.

It is helpful if the therapist can approach discussing fees in a clear, matter-of-fact manner. Some agencies offer guidelines for fee setting based upon the client's income. The term "customary and usual" is used to identify the typical fee in a particular area. Customary fees will vary based upon the geographic area. Most programs or clinicians establish a minimum fee and then work within a range. Some clinicians prefer to deal with fees in the beginning of the session when handling other administrative issues, while others feel it is best done toward the end of the initial interview.

In addition to setting the fee, you should discuss acceptable forms of payment, when the fee should be paid, and the fee for late cancellation or "no-show" appointments, if applicable. It is often useful to have a written agreement that discusses the fees and policies regarding fees. If a third party is responsible for payment, their terms for payment should be clearly understood by therapist and client. Often third-party payers limit the number of sessions, or the types of presenting problem or diagnoses they will reimburse. For example, many third-party payers will not reimburse for couple counseling or "problems of living" such as those listed in the "V" codes of the *Diagnostic and Statistical Manual of Mental Disorders* (DSM-IV-TR; American Psychiatric Association, 2000). If a third-party payer is involved, the therapist should verify insurance coverage at the outset of therapy. Issues concerning provider eligibility, annual deductible, rate of reimbursement, and limitations on the number of sessions and types of treatments covered need to be addressed. Usually a DSM-IV-TR diagnosis will need to be assigned to the insured patient.

As with other administrative issues, working out the details for payment can be part of the diagnostic process and help to clarify the family's expectations of and responsibilities for therapy. In discussing fees you might learn, for example, that a client is unable to pay the full therapy fee due to specific hardships, such as medical expenses. Alternatively, a client's unwillingness to pay the full therapy fee may reflect low motivation for therapy, a strong sense of entitlement, or a victim mentality. Generally, free services tend not to be valued by clients. A fee provides some incentive to make effective use of services.

Other Administrative Issues

Several other administrative issues need to be addressed with clients. In some cases, therapists may be required to discuss with clients their professional qualifications. For example, California law requires that all unlicensed family therapists identify themselves to their clients as trainees or interns. Many agencies and practitioners have clients read and sign an informed consent statement that generally includes a brief description of what therapy is, including the potential risks, such as being asked to examine painful issues. Informed consent statements also summarize many of the issues discussed in this chapter, such as confidentiality and payment of fees. Permission to videotape may be included in this or a separate statement. Figure 3.2 is a basic informed consent form that covers some of these issues.

DEFINING CLIENT EXPECTATIONS FOR THERAPY

Another important task in the initial interview is to define clients' expectations for what therapy will accomplish and how it will proceed, in order to ensure that clients' needs are compatible with what you, as the therapist, can or are willing to offer. In some cases, you may determine that you are not the appropriate therapist for the clients, and you will need to make a referral. In addition, clients' goals must be

I understand that treatment at _____ (name of treatment facility) may involve discussing relationship, psychological, and/or emotional issues that may at times be distressing. However, I also understand that this process is intended to help me personally and with relationships. I am aware of alternative treatment options available to me.

My therapist has satisfactorily answered all of my questions about treatment at _____ (name of treatment facility). If I have further questions, I understand that my therapist will either answer them or find answers for me. I understand that I may leave therapy at any time, although I have been informed that this is best accomplished in consultation with the therapist.

I understand that at _____ (name of treatment facility):

1. Master's or doctoral students in family therapy conduct therapy under close supervision by licensed therapists.
2. Therapy sessions are routinely videotaped and/or observed by supervisors or other therapists on the treatment team. I agree to have my sessions videotaped for the purpose of supervision or consultation with the treatment team. I understand that the videotapes are erased at the end of my treatment.

I understand that what is discussed in therapy will generally remain confidential unless I give written permission to share information from my sessions by signing a release of information. However, the therapist may share information about or videotapes of my therapy with the supervisor or treatment team in the interests of providing quality care. My therapist has also informed me that there are other possible exceptions to confidentiality, which may include, but are not limited to the following:

1. Disclosure of child abuse
2. Disclosure of elder or dependent abuse
3. Threats to harm oneself
4. Threats to harm others
5. If a court issues a subpoena
6. If you are required to be in therapy or be evaluated by a court order
7. If you claim harm to your mental or emotional state in a legal proceeding

The fee for each session will be _____, and is to be paid at the time of the therapy session. I have been informed of the cancellation policy, which states that I will pay half of the normal fee if I fail to show for the appointment or cancel a session with less than 24 hours notice.

In the event of an emergency, I have been instructed to call the Crisis Center hotline at _____ (phone number) or go to the nearest hospital emergency room.

To be signed by all participating members.

Signed: _____ Date: _____

Signed: _____ Date: _____

Signed: _____ Date: _____

Signed: _____ Date: _____

Signed: _____ Date: _____

Signed: _____ Date: _____

FIGURE 3.2. Basic informed consent form.

integrated with therapist goals to develop an effective treatment plan, which is discussed in Chapter 5.

Defining Client Goals for Therapy

The first step in defining expectations is to ask your clients what they would like to accomplish through therapy. An effective way to introduce this subject is simply to ask questions such as "How can I be helpful to you?" or "What are you hiring me to do?" Generally clients will initially respond by describing what they see as the primary problems or issues. Clients hope that you will be able to fix these problems. Individuals will often say what they want to eliminate ("I want Dad to stop nagging me") and have a harder time articulating what they want ("I want Dad to tell me I'm doing a good job"). Encourage your clients to describe desired changes in positive language (the presence of something) rather than in negative language (the absence of something).

It is important that each family member be given the opportunity to be heard when discussing problems and goals. This is obviously helpful in joining with each individual. In addition, you may discover there is disagreement about the problem itself or who has the problem. You want to give yourself the opportunity to see the problem from different perspectives, and each person will provide some information that other family members will not. An issue that can arise during this process is one family member monopolizing the conversation. It is absolutely critical that you provide enough structure to interrupt this process in order to provide space for other family members. You don't want to anger the person who talks excessively, but if you fail to interrupt this behavior the other family members may lose faith in your ability to lead the session.

In defining goals, a number of challenges can arise. Your clients may identify multiple problem areas, with little distinction of priorities. Some couples, for example, may have a "laundry list" of complaints about each other or their relationship. In these cases, you will need to obtain your clients' perspective on the relative importance of their problems. For example, you might ask, "Of the issues you have presented, which is most and which is least important?"

In other cases, your clients may not have a clear idea of what the problem is or what their goals for therapy are. In these situations you may need to contract for a limited number of sessions to explore and define problem areas and goals. Another potential problem is that clients may have unrealistically high expectations or goals. One husband, for example, expressed his belief that the couple should be totally free from any conflict after therapy. In these cases you may want to validate the client's goal and then reframe it so that it is more realistic and obtainable.

Further, setting goals may be complicated by the unstated agenda of a client, an aim that he or she feels is not appropriate to disclose. For example, a couple may come into therapy with the stated goal of working on the marriage. Later you may discover that the husband entered therapy to make sure you would take care of his wife after he informed her of his intention to leave the marriage. Sometimes, even the clients may not be totally aware of their reasons for seeking therapy. For example, a woman was eventually able to recognize that she probably was not invested in working on the relationship with her husband. Rather, she acknowledged that her motivation to try marital counseling was probably a desire to alleviate feelings of guilt about ending the marriage.

Alternatively, individuals in couples or families may define goals that initially appear incompatible. In these situations, you may need to creatively reframe the goals in such a way as to make them compatible or link them together. For example, parents may want to see their adolescent behave in a more mature and responsible manner, while the adolescent wants greater freedom. A therapist could potentially link these goals together by discussing how both the parents and adolescent have a common desire to see the adolescent become successfully launched as an adult, also pointing out that becoming an adult carries with it certain privileges as well as responsibilities. The therapist can then work with the family to help the adolescent achieve more freedom and privileges consistent with his or her ability to manage responsibility.

Another common scenario involves one partner wanting to make the relationship work, while the other individual seriously contemplates divorce. One possible approach is to suggest the need to evaluate the relationship much like a house inspector would go through a structure to determine which areas have strengths and which areas need attention. To the partner invested in the marriage, the marital evaluation could be explained as a necessary step in determining what needs to be changed if the marriage is to be saved. To the partner seriously considering divorce, the marital evaluation can be presented as a means of illuminating why this marriage failed and of helping the individual to avoid making a similar mistake in future relationships if the couple does divorce.

Once you have a clear understanding of what your clients want or expect from therapy, you need to decide whether it is appropriate for you to take on the case. First, you must assess whether the case is within your scope of practice, that is, whether the clients are expecting help for issues that would be considered appropriate for a family therapist to treat. For example, offering legal or medical advice would not be within your scope of practice, but working with a couple on their marriage obviously would be. In many cases, the scope of practice may be defined for therapists by the laws that license or certify therapists in that state. If the case falls outside your scope of practice, you will need to be able to refer your clients to an appropriate professional.

Second, you need to assess if the case falls within your scope of competence. In other words, do you have the necessary skills, training, or experience to effectively treat the issues? If not, you need to refer the clients to another therapist who has the appropriate skills or qualifications. For example, a referral would be necessary if your client wanted hypnosis but you did not have any training or experience with the technique. In some cases, you may be able to treat clients provided you take appropriate measures during treatment to gain the necessary competence. For example, a therapist who has never worked with encopresis could do a literature review on treating this condition and seek supervision on the case.

On rare occasions, the client's goals for therapy may be so incongruent with your own values that you may need to make a referral. For example, most therapists would be uncomfortable helping a client achieve the goal of convincing the partner that having extramarital affairs should be allowed in the relationship. Similarly, a pro-life therapist may have difficulty working with a client who is trying to decide whether to have an abortion.

Additional Expectations for Therapy

Many clients not only bring in expectations about what therapy will accomplish, but also about *how* therapy will do so. For example, clients who have had previous therapy may assume you will do therapy in a similar manner. If the previous therapist assigned homework, your client may also expect that of you. Whenever a client has had previous therapy, it is generally quite helpful to explore what that experience was like, as it can strongly shape (both positively and negatively) a client's expectations regarding therapy.

You need to explore with your clients what they expect to happen in therapy on a number of dimensions, including how long therapy will be and who will be involved in it. Some clients may expect therapy to be only one or two sessions, while others may expect the process to last a year or more. Likewise, an individual who expects to be seen alone may be surprised when you ask him or her to invite other family members to therapy. Clients can also have expectations about their level of involvement or that of the therapist. For example, some parents bring a troubled child to therapy with the expectation that the therapist will "fix" the child with little involvement on their part. Others expect to be an active part of the therapy process. It is critical to spell out the nature of the therapy at the outset.

You must also assess whether client expectations will impede the therapeutic process. For example, one couple stated that they did not want to look at family of origin issues since they felt this had been unproductive in previous therapy. Yet many of the couple's concerns seemed intimately tied to difficulties with their parents. In a case like this, you would need to determine how rigid the couple is in their desire to avoid family of origin exploration. If they persisted in this stance, you would have to decide how flexible you are willing to be to accommodate their desire. In some instances, you may decide against continuing therapy because the expectations are too restrictive and would severely limit your ability to be effective.

BUILDING MOTIVATION

Much of the previous discussion has assumed that clients have some voluntary interest in coming to therapy. Although many clients are motivated, you may quickly discover that not everyone willingly comes to therapy or seeks change. Some clients come to therapy because they have been mandated by the courts to do so because of substance abuse, juvenile delinquency, child abuse, or other issues. Others are forced to come to therapy by family members. A spouse may be threatened with divorce if he or she does not attend therapy; adolescents may be compelled by their parents to go to therapy. Although the therapist cannot motivate everyone, there are strategies for assessing and building motivation.

When assessing motivation, it is helpful to conceptualize it as existing on a continuum from high to low. Where clients are on the Stages of Change Cycle (Prochaska, Norcross, & DiClemente, 1994), for example, may determine their motivation for change. This cycle recognizes that clients spend a great deal of time (precontemplation and contemplation stages) thinking about changing before they decide to change and take action. In addition, the cycle recognizes that maintaining changes, such as not drinking alcohol again, can be challenging. Thus, relapse is part of the process leading to permanent change.

A client's overall level of motivation will be based on a number of factors, the assessment of which can guide you in choosing interventions that increase motivation. Motivational interviewing (Miller &

Rollnick, 2002) suggests that the therapist's job is to help the client resolve his or her ambivalence about change. Instead of using confrontation, the empathic therapist validates the client's perspective and freedom to decide. In addition, the therapist listens for the client's own self-motivation statements.

A logical time to assess motivation is when you are defining goals for therapy. Answers to the question "What brings you to therapy?" will differentiate motivated from unmotivated clients. The former usually respond by describing the problems or growth areas they would like to see addressed. If a client responds by saying that someone asked or insisted he or she come to therapy, problems with motivation may be anticipated. Nevertheless, some of these clients can become quite committed to therapy as they experience its benefits.

You should also inquire who first suggested therapy or called for the appointment. Generally this person is the most motivated for therapy. A good question to ask your clients is what led them to come to therapy now, rather than sooner or later in their lives? The answer may provide clues to your clients' motivation, as well as important assessment information, such as precipitating events.

Clients will have little motivation for therapy if they do not believe there is a problem, or if they feel that the problem is not serious. You will need to carefully assess whether a problem does indeed exist, and, if it does, why the clients refuse to acknowledge it. You may need to educate a client about the problem and the possible negative consequences of not addressing it. For example, you might warn a client that a failure to heed a partner's complaints could lead to the eventual breakup of the relationship.

Sometimes clients will deny that a problem exists out of fear of consequences or injury to their self-image. Child molesters will frequently deny or minimize the molestation to avoid legal consequences as well as to sidestep admitting to themselves that they are child molesters. In these cases, building motivation for therapy will be entwined with working with the client's denial.

If a mandated client refuses to acknowledge that a problem exists, you can suggest that there is at least one—he or she is being told to come to unwanted therapy. If your client agrees (which is typically the case), then you can explore what needs to happen so that therapy can be successfully terminated. This approach allows you to join with your client, but at the same time work on intermediate goals that address the problem.

Some clients may have poor motivation because they do not anticipate any benefit from therapy, believing that therapy is useless or the situation is hopeless. For some, creating a basis for hope will help build motivation. Noting exceptions to the problem might begin to instill some hope. Or, a positive experience in therapy during the initial session might spark hope. Of course, feelings of hopelessness and lack of motivation could be a symptom of depression. As this condition is treated through medication or other interventions, depressed clients frequently develop more energy and enthusiasm for therapy.

Other factors might also reduce clients' motivation for therapy. For example, there may be psychological barriers to therapy, such as a client having difficulty trusting others. Some clients may have practical barriers, such as difficulties with transportation, finances, or work schedules.

Using these strategies does not guarantee client motivation. You may still have a poorly motivated client, particularly in court-ordered cases in which the client can avoid prosecution by participating in therapy (for example, cases of sexual abuse or battering). In these situations, you need to become comfortable with using the leverage for change provided by the courts. For example, you may need to inform the client that therapy will be terminated and the termination reported to the courts unless satisfactory progress is maintained.

A common struggle that beginning therapists may face is when they are more motivated than their clients. At times, clients fail to show up for appointments, come late, have little to say, or do not complete their homework assignments. In these situations, the therapist may end up working much harder than the clients. This dynamic suggests that the therapist needs to step back, review the reasons for therapy, and once again evaluate the clients' motivation.

At times, clients might seem motivated "for the wrong reasons." For example, a client only quits smoking in response to a life-threatening illness. A depressed client wants to die but restrains herself because of the impact her suicide could have on her children. In couple therapy, couples may state that they are only trying to preserve their marriage "for the sake of the children." You don't need to agree with the clients' motivations. Usually, it is enough that clients, for whatever reason, will face the demanding process of change.

ESTABLISHING CREDIBILITY

Beginning therapists often fear their clients will ask, "How long have you been doing therapy?" Similarly, questions about one's marital status or parenthood may be dreaded by unmarried or childless therapists because all of these questions reflect a key issue that the beginning therapist must frequently deal with in the initial session—the issue of credibility.

In order for clients to have hope or an expectation of change, they must see the therapist and therapy as credible, or they may prematurely terminate therapy, if they begin at all. Therefore, it is important for you to assess early on any issues of credibility that need to be addressed. First, do the clients see therapy as an effective way to solve problems? Or, do they believe that therapy is only for crazy people? Second, do the clients see you, in your role as the therapist, as being competent or credible? Clients may question a therapist's ability to help them because he or she looks too young, or a parent may question a childless therapist's ability to understand and help.

If you suspect there is a credibility problem, you should attempt to pinpoint where and why credibility is lacking. For example, one beginning therapist described how a woman came into the first session saying that she wanted a gay or lesbian counselor. The therapist indicated that she was not a lesbian, and that she had very few friends who were either gay or lesbian. However, she expressed a willingness to learn more about these issues. At the end of the session, when the therapist asked how the woman felt about continuing in therapy with her, given her desire for a gay or lesbian counselor, the woman indicated she was quite comfortable about continuing with the therapist. Through further discussion, the therapist discovered that what initially had appeared to be concern about the therapist's experience working with gay or lesbian issues was actually a fear on the client's part that she would be unfairly judged by a "straight" person. When the therapist expressed an open and accepting stance toward the woman, she was able to earn the client's trust and respect. The more precise your understanding of why the client does not see you or the therapy as credible, the more likely your intervention will be on target in addressing this issue.

In cases where clients are resistant to therapy in general, you may be able to reframe the process in a way that builds its credibility. For individuals who think therapy is only for crazy people, you must work to reduce the stigma. You can compare therapy to coaching, in that even the best athletes, such as Olympians or professionals, use coaches. Therapy could also be compared to consulting work, with clients likened to businesses that hire someone with special expertise to help them.

When clients question a specific therapist's credibility, they usually focus on the lack of some critical professional or life experience. Often you can redefine for the client what type of experience is needed to be helpful. For example, a parent may doubt a therapist's ability to be helpful if he or she has not parented children of his or her own. In this instance, the therapist may be able to build credibility by discussing other types of experience working with children (e.g., taking care of a relative's children, or having been a teacher or childcare worker). Alternatively, the therapist may state that in working with several families in therapy, he or she has learned through experience what works and doesn't work in parenting.

In some cases, you can let the client know about your lack of experience in a particular area and then discuss how you can compensate for this limitation. You might indicate that your cases are supervised by a more experienced clinician, or you may ask the client to offer his or her expertise. For example, a therapist can ask clients of a different race or ethnic background to educate him or her about important cultural differences as they arise. Likewise, parents could be told that they are the experts on their children. Thus, the parents' intimate knowledge of their children plus the therapist's experience with families in general will increase the likelihood of therapy being successful.

If clients still harbor doubts, a frequently effective strategy is to contract with them for a set number of sessions (perhaps three). This gives you time to demonstrate your competence. You can explain to your clients that if they are still uncertain about your ability to help them after the agreed-upon number of sessions, you will gladly refer them elsewhere. Nearly all clients are willing to give you this chance, provided the number of sessions is reasonable. In these situations, you need to identify a problem that can be quickly resolved to build credibility with your clients.

It is important that you not become defensive if your credibility is being questioned. If you can deal with your clients' concerns in a nondefensive and respectful manner, you may actually build credibility. In order to do this, however, you must be clear in your own mind what you do have to offer, even if you have limited clinical or life experience.

First, you need to recognize that clients value having someone compassionately and respectfully listen to them at a difficult time in their lives. Part of the reason that clients' problems are so distressing to them is that they feel isolated, lonely, and inadequate in relation to others. The therapeutic relationship can provide a sense of connection and support for clients at a time when these essentials are in short supply. For some clients, the relationship with the therapist may be their first healthy relationship, and this aspect alone can be quite therapeutic. In simply being present with another human being, you have something important to offer your clients.

Second, you can frequently offer important insights to your clients because you do not have the kind of emotional involvement in the situation that they do. As an outside observer, you may help illuminate for your clients important aspects of themselves or their relationships with others that can facilitate change.

Third, even the inexperienced therapist has access to clinical knowledge that most clients do not possess or could not easily access. Through course work preparation, you have learned important concepts and theories that you may use to inform your work, thereby tapping into a source of practical knowledge and wisdom beyond your years of actual clinical experience.

CONCLUSION: THE FIRST SESSION AND BEYOND

The initial interview is a critical time in the therapy process; several important tasks must be accomplished to ensure that therapy will proceed successfully. Developing a connection and establishing credibility with your clients is essential for their return for a second session. Defining expectations for therapy and building motivation are also crucial, as well as properly handling administrative issues.

Clearly, many of the issues discussed in this chapter are important throughout therapy, not just in the first interview. You need to remain connected or joined with your clients in order to effectively confront and challenge them at all stages. Likewise, the goals or expectations for therapy may need to be redefined as therapy proceeds.

CHAPTER 4

Guidelines
for Conducting Assessment

This chapter presents a plan for approaching assessment. Beginning therapists may easily feel overwhelmed by the amount of information that needs to be gathered in the first few interviews. In an attempt to clarify the assessment process and make it less daunting, we have broken it down into various components and presented them in a logical sequence. However, the reality is that the various areas overlap, and that assessment seldom proceeds in such a straightforward manner.

Table 4.1 shows the general outline for conducting a comprehensive assessment. The initial assessment typically begins by exploring with clients their problems or concerns, and the solutions that have been attempted. At this early stage, you must also assess if your clients are in crisis, or if any possible issues of harm are relevant. For example, a client who is depressed or hopeless must be assessed for suicide. You must also be alert to possible signs of abuse or violence toward others. Since alcohol and substance abuse are commonly associated with relationship problems, they can impede effective treatment if overlooked. In addition, problems may have an underlying biological component that must be ruled out. This chapter also covers the various areas that are important to consider within a general psychosocial assessment, including assessing the individual, the couple or family system, the social systems outside the family, and larger social systems such as culture and gender socialization.

This chapter provides guidelines for conducting a comprehensive assessment within each of these areas. Such a thorough assessment will help you arrive at a more accurate picture of your client and thereby develop an effective treatment plan.

TABLE 4.1. General Assessment Plan

1. Conduct initial assessment.
   - Explore presenting problems.
   - Assess for attempted solutions.
   - Assess for crisis and stressful life events.

2. Rule out potential issues of harm.
   - Assess for suicide.
   - Assess for family violence and abuse.
   - Assess for sexual abuse.
   - Assess for duty-to-warn issues.

3. Rule out possible substance abuse.

4. Rule out possible biological problems.

5. Conduct general psychosocial assessment.
   - Assess affect, behavior, and cognitions.
   - Assess meaning system.
   - Assess spirituality.
   - Assess the couple and family system.
   - Assess social systems outside the family.
   - Assess families within the larger social context.

INITIAL ASSESSMENT

Exploring the Presenting Problems

The problems that bring clients to therapy, the presenting problems, are explored first. For example, you will want to know the nature or description of the problem—what it is, and how long it has existed. You might also inquire about who is most affected by the problem. Is it only manifested at a certain time or in a certain place? You also need to know whom the family conceptualizes as having the problem. Is the problem seen as being a relational one ("We don't know how to communicate"), or is it seen as primarily one individual's problem ("Our child is having difficulty")? When only one person is identified as having the problem, this person is often referred to as the "identified patient" or IP.

When a single IP is identified, you need to listen for and explore problems other family members may have. This has a twofold purpose. First, it helps you develop some possible hypotheses regarding family dynamics. For example, a family may initially present with a child who has problems at home or at school. With further exploration, you may discover the couple's relationship is conflictual, leading to a possible hypothesis that the child is acting out because he or she is triangulated in the couple's conflict. Second, the family is more likely to understand the justification for family therapy in lieu of individual therapy with the IP if you can successfully highlight other problems within the family system. Obviously, the more invested the family is in having an IP, the more cautiously you will need to proceed.

You should also find out who else knows about or is involved in the problem. This information can help you assess what areas of functioning have been affected by it. For example, you may learn that a child is having difficulties at school if the family discloses that a teacher knows about the problem, or you may discover that your clients are involved in the legal system. In all of these cases, you would be wise to consider getting a release of information from your clients so you can talk with others who may be knowledgeable about the problem. This can also help you assess what resources or social support the clients have. For example, a couple may mention talking to their minister or parents for advice on marital difficulties. In some cases, you may want to include some of these individuals in the treatment plan. You may solicit a teacher's help when dealing with a child's school-related problems, or parents of adult children might be invited in to deal with important family of origin issues.

Finally, it is often enlightening to ask the clients why they think the problem exists. Their insights in this area can help you develop hypotheses. It is not uncommon for one spouse to have good insights on what issues the other partner might need to look at, and vice versa. What is usually missing is insight regarding one's own issues or contributions to the problem. Likewise, ask the clients what others have said about why the problem exists. Again, this information can provide a valuable starting point for you to build hypotheses.

Some therapists who follow a solution-focused approach believe that a detailed knowledge of the problem is not always necessary to discover solutions or exceptions to the problem. Although this may indeed be true in many cases, therapists need to recognize that having clients tell us their stories (even if problem-saturated) can have value in other ways. For example, listening respectfully can help the client develop a connection with the therapist. In their eagerness to begin treatment, we have seen some beginning therapists prematurely cut off clients. Therapists need to be careful about pushing too quickly for solutions, or they risk appearing disrespectful of clients' need to tell their stories.

Assessing for Attempted Solutions

In addition to exploring the problems, it is frequently helpful to assess what solutions your clients have either attempted or considered. You thereby can avoid recommending solutions that have been unsuccessfully tried by your clients, which could damage your credibility. You should also explore what solutions your clients have considered but not tried, as well as solutions others have suggested. You can then explore with the clients why they didn't try particular solutions. This often provides you with good information about potential barriers to or negative consequences of change. Another reason to explore attempted solutions is that in some cases they may contribute to or exacerbate the problem (Fisch, Weakland, & Segal, 1985). A husband who withdraws to avoid conflict may actually create conflict with his partner because she interprets his withdrawal as a lack of caring. The therapist may recognize a pattern in a client's attempt to solve the problem and suggest that he or she take a completely different approach.

When assessing attempted solutions, it is extremely helpful to explore if therapy has been tried before. If so, you can explore what was helpful and not helpful about that experience, enabling you to build on past successes or avoid making similar mistakes. You may want to consider recommending books or giving homework assignments if your clients indicate that these were particularly helpful in the past. It would also be wise to explore why the clients are no longer seeing the previous therapist. Did the clients or therapist move, necessitating a change? Or, do your clients have a history of working with therapists a short time and then dropping out of treatment? This information will help you assess the likelihood that therapy will have a positive outcome.

Assessing for Crisis and Stressful Life Events

During the initial assessment you should assess the extent to which your clients may be in crisis. Is there a specific event bringing them into therapy, or has there been a pileup of life events that has created stress? These life events could be of a personal nature (e.g., divorce, illness, death of family member) or involve external social, economic, or political events (e.g., layoffs due to recession, immigration forced by economic or social/political hardship). Are the stressors of an acute or chronic nature? To what extent are the life stressors an underlying cause of the presenting problems? What resources do your clients have for coping? Is the stress imposing a burden on the clients that exceeds their coping resources? Whenever clients are in crisis, you should also consider assessing for suicide or other potential issues of harm. Chapter 6 discusses how to deal with clients in crisis.

POTENTIAL ISSUES OF HARM

A critical rule of assessment is the need to be constantly vigilant toward any possible issues of harm. Issues of potential harm include harm to self (suicide) or others (domestic violence or homicide, child abuse, or sexual abuse). Assessment of each of these issues is discussed herein, along with other clinical considerations.

Suicide

Research on suicide suggests that the majority of people who kill themselves have told someone about their plan in the months preceding the suicide. This person may be a family member or friend, or a physician or therapist. Family therapists work with depressed clients on a daily basis and must always be alert for signs that a client is considering suicide.

Many new therapists bring misperceptions about suicide to their first clinical experience. Two common ones are the notion that discussing thoughts of suicide may cause an attempt on the client's part, and the tendency to discount the seriousness of suicide threats, especially when others perceive them as an attempt to get attention or some other goal. Other common misperceptions include the belief that a therapist cannot intervene effectively with a client who has decided to commit suicide or that people who commit suicide really want to die.

People who kill themselves frequently are ambivalent about dying. It is usually after a series of unrelenting losses and failures, with little or no relief or hope, that a client finally chooses suicide. Even after making the decision, many suicidal people leave open a way to be rescued. For example, the writer Sylvia Plath, after several failed suicide attempts, was aware that rescue was possible from her final attempt. She turned on the gas in her stove to kill herself but knew that her maid would arrive shortly. Unfortunately, on the day of that attempt, the maid was late to work and Sylvia Plath died.

Assessing for suicide is a therapeutic skill that all beginning therapists should learn. Research has suggested there are certain demographic factors and warning signals that should alert the therapist to the possibility of client suicide attempts. Table 4.2 reflects the demographics of suicide, while Table 4.3 provides a list of danger signs that indicate suicide risk.

In assessing for suicide, the therapist may begin by simply asking the client if he or she is thinking about killing himself or herself. In listening to the client's reply, the therapist should assess (1) detail or

TABLE 4.2. Demographics of Suicide

Features	Trends and comments
Age	Suicide rises with age. The increase is linear in white males and peaks at about 50 in females. There has been a recent increase in adolescent and youth suicide.
Sex	More males commit suicide. More females attempt suicide. Recent statistics show rises in suicide rates among young white females.
Ethnicity	More whites commit suicide than nonwhites. Recent statistics show an increase in young black males ages 15–35.
Childhood loss	Early loss is associated with completed suicide, later loss with attempted suicide. Early loss is also associated with scientific and artistic creativity.
Recent loss	The more irrevocable the loss, the greater the risk of suicide. Suicide is associated with an accumulation of losses throughout life.
Alcoholism	Alcohol is associated with high risk of suicide. Treatment for drinking and suicide problems has many features in common.
Mental illness	Suicide is mostly associated with depressive illness.
Physical illness	Suicide is associated with declining health and potency.
Downward economic mobility	Unemployment, frequent job changes, and a trend toward lower status and lower-paying jobs are traditionally associated with male risk, but are no longer sex-linked characteristics.
Living in the center city	Areas of high crime, alcoholism, mental illness, poverty, and family disorganization are associated with social isolation and alienation.
Marital disruption, including divorce, widowhood, and the breaking up of a love affair	The more final the change, the more serious the risk. Marriage is more of a protection against suicide for males. Women can survive the loss of a husband better than men can survive the loss of a wife.
Previous suicide attempts	People who have attempted suicide are in a high-risk group. The more serious the previous attempts, the greater the rate of subsequent completed suicide.
History of attempted or completed suicide in relatives and other important figures	Family members' suicide is associated with a higher risk, as suicide tends to run in families.
A "death trend"	An accumulation of losses and death are a risk factor, and therefore a major reason for relieving the severe death anxiety in the family.

Note. Data from Hirschfeld and Russell (1997).

TABLE 4.3. Warning Signs of Suicide

Features	Manifestations and comments
1. Quiet, withdrawn, few friends	Often not recognized because the individual is not noticed and makes no obvious trouble. Associated with social and family isolation.
2. Changes in behavior	Personality changes, for example, from friendliness to withdrawal and lack of communication, sad and expressionless appearance; from a quiet demeanor to acting out and trouble making. The important thing is the change.
3. Increased failure or role strain	Often pervasive in school, work, home, friends, and love relationships, but often manifested most clearly in school pressures.
4. a. Recent family changes	a. Illness, job loss, increased drinking by parents or other family members. Often the background of the crisis.
b. Recent loss of a family member	b. Death, divorce, separation, or someone leaving home.
5. Feelings of despair and hopelessness	Shows itself in many forms, from changes in posture and behavior to verbal expression of such feelings. Hopelessness is even more closely associated with suicide than depression.
6. Symptomatic acts	Taking unnecessary risks, becoming involved in drinking and drug abuse, becoming inappropriately aggressive or submissive. Giving away possessions. Associated with changes in behavior.
7. Communication of suicidal thoughts or feelings	Such statements as "Life is not worth living," "I'm finished," "Done for," "I might as well be dead," or "I wish I was dead." Best understood in the context of life changes and family changes.
8. Presence of a plan	Storing up medication, buying a gun. The meaning of these acts and communication can best be understood by sensitive responding to and questioning of the suicidal person.
9. Negative or fearful attitudes toward treatment or psychiatrists	"Shows you're crazy," "It's the end of the road," "I'll end up in the crazy house," and so on. Refusal of help. Associated with conflicts over family loyalties.
10. Impasse in therapy	"Sabotaging" of the therapy, extreme resistance, becoming increasingly depressed or suicidal. Known as the "negative therapeutic reaction," it is often associated with success in therapy and threats to the status quo. Also part of a potentially positive therapeutic crisis.

Note. Data from Hirschfeld and Russell (1997).

specificity in the plan (is there mention of a method, time and date, or a planned or written suicide note?); (2) lethality and reversibility (e.g., shooting vs. cutting oneself); (3) intentionality (providing for the possibility of rescue); and (4) proximity (whether important support people know of the plan, are nearby, and express care or concern for the client). The therapist should also assess the same factors in any previous suicide attempts. Additional risk factors include psychiatric diagnosis, antisocial or borderline personality disorders, substance use, sense of urgency, poor impulse control, poor reality testing, serious medical illness, and life stress.

In addition, the assessment should examine or discover what would prevent the person from committing suicide. In essence, the therapist wants to know what would give the person hope. For example, a divorced, unemployed woman stated that the only reason she did not commit suicide was the pain it would cause her children. The therapist realized that the client was in so much pain that no amount of talk about caring for herself would change her mind. However, her sense of duty and love for her children combined with her religious beliefs about suicide served as strong enough deterrents to keep her alive until her living situation improved. Therapists can listen to and reinforce reasons their clients have for not killing themselves.

Discussing the suicidal ideation or suicide attempts of an individual in front of other family members involves important considerations. The therapist should determine what role family members may serve in preventing or increasing the possibility of a member attempting suicide. For example, family members sometimes threaten suicide when they perceive the possibility of rejection or abandonment by another family member (as in divorce). Intense family conflict can be the precipitating event in an adolescent's suicide attempt. On the other hand, the desire to protect young children from harm can be the only reason a parent stays alive. One client family lost a 16-year-old son in a skiing accident, causing the mother to go into a deep depression. Two years later the mother reported that the only factor that kept her from a suicide attempt was the desire to protect her 12-year-old daughter from further loss.

The possibility of suicide is often an unstated family secret of which members are aware in varying degrees. Depending on the age, maturity, and relationships of family members, an open discussion of suicide can lift a burden off the family. Social isolation, family history of suicide attempts, and loss of family members through death or separation are predictors of suicide that specifically involve family relations. Relationships among family members are an important consideration in any discussion of suicide.

Assessing for Violence and Abuse

Estimates of family violence suggest that some type of violence occurs in approximately 15–20% of families. Violence can take many forms and be inflicted in many different relationships. While spousal abuse and physical abuse of children are probably the most common forms of violence that therapists see, violence against the elderly is becoming increasingly common. Victims of family violence can suffer a wide range of physical and psychological problems. Battering, for example, is the most common cause of injury for women.

It is recommended that you routinely evaluate all couples for domestic violence (Riggs, Caulfield, & Street, 2000). One way to uncover domestic violence is to ask couples to describe what an argument or fight looks like. It may be necessary to ask directly if one or both individuals has ever hit, harmed, or threatened his or her partner. Some individuals may be reluctant to admit in front of their partner that there has been domestic violence out of a fear that this will lead to violence at home after the therapy session. As a result, some clients will not admit to any domestic violence unless asked in an individual session. The clinician should suspect domestic violence if an individual has sustained injuries and does not offer a plausible explanation for them. Assessment measures such as the Conflict Tactics Scale (Straus, 1979) can also be used to screen for possible intimate partner violence.

While many warning signs may suggest that some type of violence is occurring, therapists should also pay attention to their internal responses to the clients. Frequently, students report having a nagging concern about a family member's safety, even when the session is over. Another frequent internal clue is the therapist's sense of fearfulness, intimidation, and concern for personal safety, particularly because many beginning therapists are young and female.

There is increasing evidence that there are different types of domestic violence (Greene & Bogo, 2002). In one type of violence ("patriarchal terrorism"), the perpetrator uses violence to exert control over the partner. Men are most likely to be the perpetrator in this type of domestic violence. In the second type of violence ("common couple violence"), partners intermittently become physical with one another when an argument escalates. In contrast to the first type, this type of violence is not characterized by a pervasive pattern of control, and may be initiated by either partner. Regardless of the type, it is important that the therapist take the violence seriously and insist that it stop.

Greene and Bogo (2002) suggest four factors that may help clinicians distinguish between patriarchal terrorism and common couple violence. In contrast to common couple violence, the perpetrator in patriarchal terrorism uses a variety of control tactics besides violence, including emotional abuse, isolation, threats, and control of finances or other resources. Second, the motivation for violence is different. In patriarchal terrorism, the goal is to establish control over one's partner, which is not true for common couple violence. Third, the impact is usually more severe in patriarchal terrorism, often because the type of violence is more severe. Physical and emotional well-being, occupational functioning, and relationships with those outside the couple (e.g., friends, family) are more likely to be affected if the individual is suffering from patriarchal terrorism. Finally, the individual's subjective experience of the violence may be different. In common couple violence, individuals may not fear their partner, whereas this is almost always the case in patriarchal terrorism.

Distinguishing between these two types of domestic violence is important because it can have implications for treatment. It may be feasible, for example, to conduct conjoint couple therapy with common couple violence. However, this type of treatment would be contraindicated when the partner engages in patriarchal terrorism. Rather, treatment for the perpetrator focuses on addressing male power and control. Emotional dependence and lack of economic options are two reasons women stay in relationships where there is battering or patriarchal terrorism. This situation has led to treatment ideas that focus on finding shelter, economic options, and new connections to supportive people and resources for victims.

Although society and the legal system historically have been slower to intervene in violence between two adults, they have been more attentive to cases that involve potential child abuse. This heightened responsiveness to child abuse is most likely in response to the fact that children are less powerful and able to protect themselves than adults. Frequently, domestic violence and child abuse occur in the same families and are perpetrated by a man who was abused himself as a child. Additional predictors of abuse are families who suffer economic hardships and who are isolated from outside support systems.

Although some children will disclose directly (often privately) an incidence of physical abuse, others will not. Physical abuse should be suspected if children give evasive or unconvincing stories as to how they obtained their injuries (e.g., bruises, burns, welts, broken bones). When asked about how they discipline their children, parents may disclose examples of physical abuse, but may either not recognize it as abuse or justify the behavior (e.g., as necessary to get the child to behave).

Therapists also need to be alert to possible neglect, another form of child abuse. Children who suffer from neglect may wear clothing that is dirty, ill-fitting, or inappropriate for the weather. They may also be consistently dirty or have severe body odor. A home that is dirty or severely cluttered may be evidence of neglect. Neglect should also be suspected if children receive inadequate medical or dental care, or are left home alone without proper supervision. You should carefully assess for neglect if parents are severely depressed or using substances since this may impact their ability to provide for their children.

As with violence, sexual abuse occurs more frequently than reported. The definition of sexual abuse varies from state to state, but usually it is said to occur when an adult or older child initiates an interaction with a child for the purpose of sexually stimulating or gratifying the perpetrator. Although research varies, national surveys indicate that approximately one in five women and one in nine men report being victims of sexual abuse as children (Finkelhor, Hotaling, Lewis, & Smith, 1990). The majority of sexual abuse cases involve male perpetrators and female victims.

Perpetrators and victims of childhood sexual maltreatment usually do not voluntarily self-report; detection is often left to the therapist, who may be given indirect behaviors as clues. Due to the legal implications of both physical and sexual abuse, it is vital to handle each case with care, since specific court testimony might be needed. Limiting the number of times a child discloses his or her experience is vital for the emotional welfare of the child.

Using a biopsychosocial perspective, sexual abuse assessment stems from information about a child's physical condition, behavior, and social context. If a child indicates several of the following symptoms, further interviewing needs to be done: (1) physically, a child may display sleep disturbances, encopresis, or enuresis, complain of abdominal pain, or suffer from appetite disturbances with corresponding weight change; (2) behaviorally, a child may manifest a sudden, unexplained change in behavior (anxiety or depression), regressive behavior, or overly sexualized behavior or knowledge given the child's age, experience suicidal thoughts, run away, or abuse substances; (3) socially, family conditions may include a child's parentified role, inadequate parental coping skills, marital difficulties leading to one parent seeking physical affection from the child, isolated social context, alcohol and drug use, and a history of parental sexual abuse (Edwards & Gil, 1986).

Child sexual abuse can negatively impact individuals in a number of ways, including risk of posttraumatic stress disorder, depression, suicide, and sexual promiscuity (Paolucci, Genius, & Violato, 2001). Survivors of child sexual abuse can also experience problems later on in their intimate relationships as result of the abuse, including issues with sexual functioning (Davis & Petretic-Jackson, 2000; Rumstein-McKean & Hunsley, 2001). Multiple factors such as the duration and severity of the abuse can influence the effects on the victim. The family response to the disclosure of sexual abuse can also mediate the impact of the abuse. Families that believe the child's claims of sexual abuse and take appropriate action to protect the child from further abuse can aid in the child's healing. In contrast, a family that does not believe the child or blames the child for the abuse can add to the child's victimization. In many cases, victims of child sexual abuse misplace blame on themselves for the abuse, which increases their sense of shame. If sexual abuse is uncovered, you should carefully assess what effect the abuse has had on the individual and factors that may mediate its impact.

When working with the elderly or families with dependent adults, you should also be alert to the possibility of abuse or neglect. Elder or dependent adults may tell you directly about possible abuse, which can take many forms, such as physical abuse, sexual abuse, neglect, or financial abuse. Like other forms of family violence or abuse, you may need to ask directly if the individual has experienced any form of violence, abuse, or neglect, especially if you have any suspicions. Unexplained injuries such as bruising or marks, for example, should be inquired about. Caretakers can be asked how they deal with the elder or dependent individual when they are frustrated. You should also be attentive to possible signs of neglect, such as the individual not being properly groomed, or not receiving appropriate care for medical or physical needs.

Legal issues are an important concern when either violence or abuse is suspected or known. In most states, the law mandates the reporting of physical abuse, neglect, or sexual abuse of children. Reporting of elder or dependent abuse may also be mandated. Except in *Tarasoff* or "duty to warn" situations (see below), therapists may have no legal responsibility to report domestic violence. It is imperative that you know the laws of your state in this regard.

Beyond legal knowledge, one's best clinical judgment will be required in some situations. For example, in most states mandated reporters (which usually include therapists) are required to report *suspected* abuse. Therapists are given significant power by the law surrounding abuse issues. Several lawsuits have been initiated by family members who have been accused of abuse that they assert they did not commit. This is especially problematic when the victim is older and the accusations are based on repressed memories that have surfaced in therapy. Suspicions about abuse in a particular family can change the family's life irrevocably. What constitutes enough evidence to report requires judgment that most beginning therapists are still developing.

When new therapists initially suspect abuse, they should immediately involve their supervisors.

Gathering information is another skill that therapists develop over time. Particularly when abuse is suspected, the therapist must be careful in eliciting and documenting information. Ideally, the interview could be on videotape, carried out with a supervisor or more experienced therapist. The therapist wants to know the who, what, how, where, and why of each situation without asking leading questions or giving responses that might influence what the victim says. The therapist also needs to assess for imminent risk. Interviewing possible child abuse victims is an art requiring specialized training and skill development. If child abuse is suspected, the family therapist will continue to interview if trained to do so, or will refer the child to a specialist, usually through child protective services available in the community.

When violence or abuse is an issue, the therapist can no longer conduct "therapy as usual." Insight into the violence will not protect the victims. Safety of the victims at home and during the therapy sessions is of paramount importance. This means that the therapist must become very practical in his or her treatment approach, finding out if the victims can escape and if they have a safe place to go. If the victims are children or elderly and thus unable to protect themselves, the therapist must be even more active, becoming a representative of society by stating unequivocally that the violence must stop immediately and then notifying the proper authorities to ensure that it does.

The switch from client's advocate exploring therapeutic issues or assessing and addressing practical concerns of living and safety to representative of society using one's authority to stop a client's behavior can be a difficult process for beginning therapists. Most therapists choose their profession because they want to help people in a collaborative manner. Violence and abuse are two of the infrequent therapeutic situations in which therapists must take an authoritarian stance and insist that a behavior stop.

Duty-to-Warn Issues

Another potential safety issue therapists may encounter is a client who threatens to kill or harm another. A psychologist at a university counseling center faced one such situation when his client Prosenjit Poddar threatened to kill his girlfriend. The therapist notified campus police, who questioned and released Prosenjit. Two months later, Prosenjit killed his girlfriend, Tatiana Tarasoff. The courts (*Tarasoff v. Regents of the University of California*) later ruled that the psychologist had not taken sufficient action to prevent the harm because he did not notify Tatiana Tarasoff of the threat. As a result of this case, many states require therapists to inform potential victims if a serious threat has been made against them, referred to as a duty-to-warn. You must learn the laws in your own state regarding when a "duty to warn" situation exists and what actions are required from you. In California, for example, therapists are mandated to warn identifiable potential victims and contact law enforcement to obtain legal immunity.

In identifying the seriousness of the risk, several factors should be considered. Borum and Reddy (2001) have suggested six factors that clinicians can use, which together form the acronym ACTION. The first factor is to explore "Attitudes that support or facilitate violence." For example, does the client believe that violence is justified in certain situations or circumstances? C refers to "Capacity." Does the client have access to the means (e.g., weapons) to carry out the threats? Does the client have access to the individual or individuals that he or she is threatening to harm? The letter T represents "Thresholds crossed," which encourages the therapist to find out if the client has a plan, and the extent to which he or she has begun to put a plan into action. Therapists should also assess for "Intent." Does a client's comment reveal a serious intent to harm others, or is it a general comment that reflects frustration but no serious intention of harming another? O stands for "Others' reactions and responses." Have others, for example, encouraged or discouraged the individual with regard to acting in a hostile way? "Noncompliance with risk reduction" is the last factor. Risk is higher if the individual shows an unwillingness to consider alternatives to harming others. In addition to the above factors, it is important to assess if the client has a previous history of violence toward others, or has a mental illness that would predispose him or her to violence.

ASSESSING FOR SUBSTANCE ABUSE

Substance abuse is one of the major mental health problems in the United States. In fact, many healthcare payer groups single out substance abuse as a separate budget item. Although some experts assert that there is a substance abuse epidemic, abuse and addictions are commonly overlooked in therapy unless the substance problem is the presenting problem.

Therapists overlook substance abuse issues for a variety of reasons. First, the clients may not consider the abuse to be a problem itself, but, rather, the result of some other issue: a bad job, painful childhood, or conflictual marriage. Clients come to therapy asking for help with the presenting problem and fail to mention their substance abuse. The therapist might collude by failing to ask about use of substances, or drug and alcohol abuse might be overlooked because there is no clear definition of when a social drinker becomes a problem drinker or when the latter becomes an alcoholic. In other words, the abuser might not view his or her substance use as problematic. The family may consider the substance use a problem but be afraid to mention it.

One of the authors had a client family report that the father could not be an alcoholic because he only drank beer. Families have different definitions about what constitutes a substance abuse problem. Is dependence on caffeine an addiction? Is recreational use of marijuana a problem? When does regular substance use become a problem? Experts do not agree on these issues, and neither do families. Even if families believe that a member's substance abuse is a problem, they often collude to hide it from the therapist.

For example, a therapist had as clients a couple who defined the wife's presenting problem as the husband's drinking. The husband's presenting problem was the wife's nagging, particularly about his drinking. The therapist presented the following three theories to the couple and suggested that the goal of therapy was to decide which theory was true: (1) alcohol abuse by the husband was the problem; (2) conflict about the alcohol was the problem in the relationship; or (3) the wife's distortions about the alcohol were the problem. He then challenged the husband to quit drinking for 2 weeks to help discern "the truth." When the husband could not quit drinking, he became willing to consider the first theory.

The most common mistake new therapists make regarding substance abuse is to overlook the possibility of it. Substance abuse is frequently comorbid with, that is, it exists along with, other disorders such as depression or anxiety. It also is associated with violence, abuse, automobile accidents, homicides, and suicide. It is essential to know the variety of ways substance-abusing clients can present in therapy. The second step is to routinely ask about substance use in initial interviews with new clients.

There are several commonly used screening tests for assessing alcohol abuse (Kitchens, 1994). Questions raised in these tests can be asked about substances other than alcohol. Two frequently used tests are the Michigan Alcoholism Screening Test (MAST) and the Alcohol Use Disorders Identification Test (AUDIT), depicted in Figures 4.1 and 4.2, respectively. The MAST has been widely used and has been examined with generally favorable results in terms of reliability and accuracy. It is made up of 24 yes/no questions and scoring indicates the subject's degree of alcohol dependence. Shorter versions of the MAST

Points	Questions
2	1. Do you feel you are a normal drinker?
2	2. Have you ever awakened the morning after some drinking the night before and found that you could not remember a part of the evening before?
1	3. Does your spouse or do your parents ever worry or complain about your drinking?
2	4. Can you stop drinking without a struggle after one or two drinks?
1	5. Do you ever feel bad about your drinking?
2	6. Do friends or relatives think you are a normal drinker?
2	7. Are you always able to stop drinking when you want to?
5	8. Have you ever attended a meeting of Alcoholics Anonymous?
1	9. Have you gotten into fights when drinking?
2	10. Has drinking ever created problems with you and your spouse?
2	11. Has your spouse or other family member ever gone to anyone for help about your drinking?
2	12. Have you ever lost friends or girlfriends/boyfriends because of your drinking?
2	13. Have you ever gotten into trouble at work because of drinking?
2	14. Have you ever lost a job because of drinking?
2	15. Have you ever neglected your obligations, your family, or your work for two or more days in a row because you were drinking?
1	16. Do you ever drink before noon?
2	17. Have you ever been told you have liver trouble? Cirrhosis?
2	18. Have you ever had delirium tremens (DTs) or severe shaking, heard voices, or seen things that weren't there after heavy drinking?
5	19. Have you ever gone to anyone for help about your drinking?
5	20. Have you ever been in a hospital because of your drinking?
2	21. Have you ever been a patient in a psychiatric hospital or on a psychiatric ward of a general hospital where drinking was part of the problem?
2	22. Have you ever been seen at a psychiatric or mental health clinic or gone to a doctor, social worker, or clergyman for help with an emotional problem in which drinking had played a part?
2	23. Have you ever been arrested, even for a few hours, because of drunken behavior?
2	24. Have you ever been arrested for drunk driving or driving after drinking?

FIGURE 4.1. Michigan Alcoholism Screening Test (MAST). From Selzer (1971). Copyright 1971 by the American Psychiatric Association. Reprinted by permission.

have also been developed. The AUDIT questionnaire is much shorter but has less data on reliability and validity.

The CAGE (Cutting down, Annoying, Guilt, Eye-opener) questionnaire (Ewing, 1984) consists of four questions: (1) Have you ever felt you ought to cut down on your drinking? (2) Have people annoyed you by criticizing your drinking? (3) Have you ever felt bad or guilty about your drinking? (4) Have you ever had a drink first thing in the morning to steady your nerves or get rid of a hangover (an eye-opener)? These simple questions can be memorized and integrated with a regular intake interview.

The CAGE questionnaire has been tested for accuracy in several different settings. Generally, a positive response to two or more questions identifies a problem drinker. Frequency is another key variable in the assessment of a substance problem. Other behaviors that might indicate a substance problem include the amount of substance used in one setting, the reasons the client uses the substance, and what happens when the client tries to stop using the substance.

ASSESSING FOR BIOLOGICAL AND NEUROLOGICAL FACTORS

George Gershwin spent several years in psychoanalysis with an analyst who had two medical degrees. When he finally died, an autopsy found a brain tumor that explained his aberrant behavior. To avoid making the same mistake as Gershwin's analyst, family therapists must consider biological or organic factors in assessment. Unfortunately, the reality is that family therapists are trained to recognize and treat psychological and social problems and frequently have limited knowledge of biological influences on behavior. Thus, we run the risk of misinterpreting important clues to a possible biological problem as a symptom of something we have been trained to treat—interpersonal problems. However, being mindful of this risk can help keep us from overlooking possible biological or organic factors.

An awareness of biological problems does not require that you be an expert in human physiology. However, therapists must recognize the telltale signs of an underlying biological problem and also recognize that psychological symptoms do not necessarily imply psychological causes (Taylor, 1990). You also need sensitivity to any information that seems outside the usual content of a family therapy session. Instead of dismissing the unusual content because it does not fit with one's model, a therapist needs an attitude of openness and curiosity to pursue a line of questioning wherever it may lead, including to a referral.

1. How often do you have a drink containing alcohol?

| Never | Monthly or less | 2 to 4 times a month | 2 or 3 times a week | 4 or more times a week |

2. How many drinks containing alcohol do you have on a typical day when you are drinking?

| 1 or 2 | 3 or 4 | 5 or 6 | 7 to 9 | 10 or more |

3. How often do you have 6 or more drinks on one occasion?

| Never | Less than monthly | Monthly | Weekly | Daily or almost daily |

4. How often during the last year have you found that you were not able to stop drinking once you had started?

| Never | Less than monthly | Monthly | Weekly | Daily or almost daily |

5. How often during the last year have you failed to do what was expected from you because of drinking?

| Never | Less than monthly | Monthly | Weekly | Daily or almost daily |

6. How often during the last year have you needed a first drink in the morning to get yourself going after a heavy drinking session?

| Never | Less than monthly | Monthly | Weekly | Daily or almost daily |

7. How often in the last year have you had a feeling of guilt or remorse after drinking?

| Never | Less than monthly | Monthly | Weekly | Daily or almost daily |

8. How often during the last year have you been unable to remember what happened the night before because you had been drinking?

| Never | Less than monthly | Monthly | Weekly | Daily or almost daily |

9. Have you or someone else been injured as a result of your drinking?

| No | Yes, but not in the last year | Yes, during the last year |

10. Has a relative or friend or a doctor or other health worker been concerned about your drinking or suggested you cut down?

| No | Yes, but not in the last year | Yes, during the last year |

FIGURE 4.2. Alcohol Use Disorders Identification Test (AUDIT). From Saunders, Aasland, Babor, De La Fuente, and Grant (1993). Copyright 1993 by the Society for the Study of Addiction to Alcohol and Other Drugs, Carfax Publishing Ltd., Abingdon, UK. Reprinted by permission of Blackwell Publishing Ltd.

Therapists should be aware of several clues that might indicate biological problems, including (1) no history of similar symptoms; (2) no readily identifiable cause; (3) age 55 or older; (4) chronic physical disease; and (5) drug use. Some clues in particular suggest the possibility of organic brain disease. Symptoms of a brain disease might result from a brain tumor, seizures, heart disease, or liver failure. One or more of the following cognitive deficits suggest a brain syndrome: inattention, disorientation, recent memory impairment, diminished reasoning, and sensory indiscrimination. Other clues suggesting a brain syndrome include head injury, changes in headache pattern, visual disturbances, speech deficits, abnormal body movements, and alterations in consciousness. The more clues there are, the more suspicious you should be. These clues should alert you to begin a different line of questioning, focusing on the individual and his or her symptoms. Other family members may be asked to corroborate details given by the IP or to give their own impressions. Discovery of these symptoms should lead you to make a prompt referral for medical evaluation. Document this referral in the client's record and note the reasons the referral was made.

An important diagnostic tool that family therapists should be familiar with is the mental status exam (MSE). MSEs are used frequently by physicians during physical exams as a rapid assessment tool to detect changes in orientation, intellectual functioning (language, memory, and calculation), thought content, judgment, mood, and behavior. MSEs are used less frequently in family therapy, perhaps because most clients who come for family treatment do not demonstrate any behaviors that would raise concerns about intellectual functioning.

While it is probably prudent to refer a client to a physician if unusual symptoms (such as those listed earlier) are noted, you can conduct an MSE immediately and obtain information that will be helpful in making a referral. When doing an MSE, the therapist should consider the client's appearance; his or her interaction with others; the client's awareness of where he or she is and what he or she is doing; appropriateness of behavior; the client's mood, use of language, attention, and concentration; short- and long-term memory; ability to perform simple calculations and answer specific questions; the presence of delusions (bizarre thoughts) with or without hallucinations; social and moral judgment; and impulsiveness (Dilsaver, 1990). Figure 4.3 provides a sample of the factors considered during a thorough MSE, while Figure 4.4 includes a number of questions that can be asked in a brief mental status check.

A short mnemonic to remember the elements of an MSE is JOIMAT: judgment, orientation, intellectual functioning, memory, affect, and thought processing. A family therapist may perform MSEs so infre-

1. Is the client's appearance unusual?

2. Is the nature and quality of the client's interaction with the examining therapist and others (such as family members or friends) appropriate?

3. Is the client oriented to person, place, and time (orientation to time includes the ability to specify the month, the day of the month, the day of the week, the year, and the season of the year)?

4. Is the client oriented to the circumstances? Does the client understand the nature of the therapist/client relationship and have an appropriate manner?

5. What is the client's affect (predominant emotional tone)?

6. What is the client's mood (reported emotional state)? Is the reported mood congruent with therapist's perception of affect?

7. Is there evidence of an abnormality in the sphere of language? Consider rate, intonation, modulation, nonverbal gestures and expressions, and whether these are congruent with content. Is there evidence of aphasia?

8. Is the content of the client's thought noteworthy? Is there evidence of delusions, obsessions, or unnecessary worry or phobias?

9. Is there abnormality in any of the five senses? Are there reports of hallucinations or delusions?

10. Are the client's attention and concentration impaired?

11. Are defects in short- or long-term memory reported or detected on formal examination of these abilities?

12. Is the client's social and moral judgment within the limits of his or her cultural group?

13. Does the client have suicidal or homicidal ideation or intent? Does the client have the means to carry out any plans to harm self or others? What is the client's level of impulse control?

14. Can the client perform calculations with the speed and accuracy expected of someone with the same educational and occupational background?

15. Is the client properly oriented in space? Does the client distinguish between right and left?

16. Does the client have the sense of direction that is expected? (Are there reports of getting lost when traveling repeated routes?)

17. Is the client's ability to think abstractly commensurate with his or her educational background?

18. Can the client copy geometric figures?

FIGURE 4.3. Some factors considered during a mental status exam. Adapted from Dilsaver (1990). Copyright 1990 by the American Academy of Family Physicians. Adapted by permission.

1. What is the date today?
2. What day of the week is it?
3. What is the name of this place?
4. What is your telephone number (or address)?
5. How old are you?
6. When were you born?
7. Who is the President of the United States now?
8. Who was the President just before that?
9. What was your mother's maiden name?
10. Subtract 3 from 20 and keep subtracting 3 from each new number you get, all the way down.

For clients with high school education:

0–2 errors = intact mental function
3–4 errors = mild mental impairment
5–7 errors = moderate mental impairment
8–10 errors = severe mental impairment

Allow one more error if the client has only a grade school education. Allow one less error if the client has education beyond high school.

FIGURE 4.4. Short Mental Status Questionnaire. Adapted from Dilsaver (1990) and Pfeiffer (1975). Copyrights 1990 by the American Academy of Family Physicians and 1975 by the American Geriatrics Society/Wiley Periodicals, Inc. Adapted by permission.

quently that it is difficult to remember the details of the exam. However, by memorizing the mnemonic and asking oneself, "What is unusual about this client and what questions should I ask to obtain more information?" you can begin investigating possible biological etiologies. For example, an elderly couple was receiving supportive family therapy in conjunction with the husband's treatment for lung cancer, which was in remission. During one session, the husband seemed confused and unable to focus. The therapist wondered if these behaviors were cognitive symptoms of depression, which is a normal response to cancer. However, the therapist referred the husband back to his physician, and a CT scan was done, with the results indicating that the cancer had spread to his brain.

In general, a family therapist might consider requesting a neuropsychological evaluation when the following problems emerge: learning problems in children or adults, memory problems, language struggles, and organizational struggles with planning or completing tasks. If a client's daily functioning changes dramatically at school or work, the therapist can consider requesting a neuropsychological evaluation. For neuropsychological evaluations, young clients and elderly clients are the most commonly referred patients. Young clients who struggle at school might have learning disabilities. The elderly might have dementia, delirium, or depression. A neuropsychological evaluation can help tease out the reasons for the client's struggles and suggest a direction for treatment.

In general, neuropsychiatric testing evaluates intellectual functioning, attention, decision making, memory, visual-spatial skills, language, motor functioning, and emotional functioning. Most evaluations are done by neuropsychologists with PhDs. However, school psychologists can also do evaluations, and these are less costly. For the elderly, a neurologist or psychiatrist would probably do the evaluation. Family therapists often treat families with the presenting complaint of a child's "laziness," "attitude problem," or "defiance." In fact, the child might have a known syndrome such as ADHD. A wonderful opportunity exists for family therapists to help their client families understand how a child's brain works and what the child needs to prosper and learn. A good neuropsychological exam can provide new understanding of the child's struggles. The family therapist can reframe the problem and provide insight into the child's unique learning style. In like manner, using the results of a neuropsychological evaluation, a family therapist can help a family understand the unique needs of an elderly family member. These skills will be especially important as the general population continues to age.

GENERAL PSYCHOSOCIAL ASSESSMENT

Psychopathology and the ABCs: Assessing Affect, Behavior, and Cognition

Most psychological theories focus on affect, behaviors, or cognitions. As a result, both assessment and treatment goals usually address one of these domains. We believe that all good clinicians attend to affect, behavior, and cognitions regardless of their theoretical orientation. A key reason to assess all three domains is that symptom descriptions for mental disorders in DSM-IV-TR usually fall into one of these categories.

Certain disorders of childhood, such as oppositional defiant disorder and conduct disorder, focus almost exclusively on behaviors, while delusional disorder focuses on patients' beliefs about themselves or their relationships, and mood disorders primarily involve changes in emotion and affect. Symptom lists for most DSM-IV-TR disorders address all three domains, although the focus varies by disorder. In recent years, DSM editors have tried to remove the theory-driven terminology (e.g., such phrases as "defense mechanisms") and instead use observable criteria. These changes should make it easier to do an assessment of the patient's symptoms.

During your assessment, consider whether the problems the client describes and those you observe fit more into one category than another. You can consider the "ABCs" as well as whether the symptoms cluster together in a way that matches a DSM-IV-TR diagnosis, although family systems theory usually describes interaction, not individual symptoms (Denton, Patterson, & Van Meir, 1997). It is not necessary to be a purist, choosing an exclusive focus on family interaction or individual diagnosis—using both frameworks can lead to the most complete assessment picture.

It is important that you have a basic understanding of DSM-IV-TR because it represents the common language shared by mental health clinicians. In addition, many treatment methods and psychopharmacological remedies are tied to DSM-IV-TR individual diagnostic categories. While you may not have memorized criteria for every possible diagnosis, you should be able to recognize depression, anxiety, substance abuse, somatization, and other common disorders. Cultivate an attitude of curiosity, and think of yourself as a keen observer of the human condition. Write down a list of the most salient symptoms your patient describes, and note your own observations along with the nature of your interaction with the client. Then ask yourself, do these symptoms cluster in a way that fits a DSM-IV-TR diagnostic category? Consider also the possibility that your patient may demonstrate more than one disorder; comorbidity is common.

Assessing for Meaning

One of the most important aspects of assessment is to understand the meaning system that each client attaches to the issues presented in therapy. The meaning system is essentially composed of the various cognitions, beliefs, memories, and emotions that a client consciously or unconsciously uses to make sense of his or her daily experiences. The meaning system influences how the individual views and interprets internal and external experiences, and how he or she chooses to respond to those experiences.

It will be difficult for you to create change without understanding how your clients make meaning out of their experiences. In one case, a woman with a chronic illness became upset whenever her husband offered any type of advice regarding her illness. She accused him of being very unsupportive of her and her illness, and was threatening to leave the relationship. He in turn was hurt and confused by this accusation because he felt he was expressing concern whenever he suggested things to her. By exploring the meaning that the woman ascribed to her husband's advice giving, the therapist discovered that she interpreted his advice as evidence that he thought her chronic illness could be cured. She feared that once he truly discovered that her illness was chronic and not curable, he would perceive her as a burden and leave. This opened the door to discussing important issues in the relationship regarding illness, caretaking, and trust.

You can use a variety of approaches to understanding or map the client's meaning system. Usually the best approach is to ask your client directly what meaning he or she attributes to something. However, this approach is not infallible. In order to trust your client's self-report, you must have confidence that your client is being honest, is cooperative, and is sufficiently self-aware. Clients are not always willing or capable of this. For example, child molesters may be unwilling to fully disclose details or even admit to molesting a child out of shame or fear of legal consequences. In some cases, clients may have little psychological insight into their motives or reasons for doing things. To the extent that we all have some psychological processes that operate outside of our immediate awareness, client self-report has some limitations.

In addition to self-reports, you can sometimes infer aspects of your client's meaning system based on his or her observable behavior and the context in which that behavior happens. When a husband silently withdraws after his wife criticizes him, the inference can be made that the husband was hurt by the remark. The difficulty with making inferences based on behaviors is that several alternate meanings are possible, raising the possibility that an incorrect inference will be made. This risk is evident when working with distressed couples; clients frequently attribute a more negative intent to their partner's behavior than the partner intended.

Your knowledge in specific content areas can also be an important aid in inferring how information is processed by each individual. For example, a good grounding in human development can help you understand an adolescent's behavior in the context of his or her need for independence. Likewise, understanding a client's cultural background may provide important insights when an individual's interpretations of certain behaviors or events differ from those common in the dominant culture.

Assessing Spirituality

One of the most crucial areas that therapists often overlook in their assessment of meaning is the client's religious or spiritual life (Bergin, 1991). Therapists have been reluctant to address spiritual issues for several reasons. One is that many therapists were trained during a time when the scientific-empirical epistemology was held in high esteem. During their training, therapists learned that if it can't be measured, it shouldn't be considered in assessment. In addition, conducting an assessment implies the possibility of treatment. Most therapists would consider themselves unable to provide spiritual solutions or treatment and would perhaps equate any spiritual treatment as a form of proselytizing.

Bergin (1991) encourages psychotherapists to consider spiritual issues as part of psychotherapy by noting that a spiritual perspective can strongly contribute to a client's (and therapist's) view of human nature, morality, and religious rituals and practices. In addition, he points out that therapists' lack of recognition of religious and spiritual practices is largely at odds with the beliefs of the clients they treat. The general public is more religious, and more prone to rely on religious tenets, than psychotherapists are (Bergin, 1991). For example, a Gallup poll found that 50% of elderly people surveyed said they wanted their doctors to pray with them as they faced death, and 75% said that physicians (and therapists) should address spiritual issues as part of their care (Connell, 1995).

When assessing spiritual issues, you can conceptualize your role as one of asking open-ended questions, assuming a position of curiosity about your client's beliefs, and seeking simply to understand your client's story (Griffith & Griffith, 1994). For example, you can ask yourself, "In what ways and for how long has this patient's life been changed as a result of spiritual beliefs and experiences?" The spiritual experience need not be dramatic for a genuine "conversion" in terms of a changed life to occur.

Several models for spiritual assessment and research instruments have been developed in the last 20 years (Fitchett, 1993). Fitchett's 7×7 model for spiritual assessment is one example of such an assessment guide (see Figure 4.5). Many of these models focus on understanding how spiritual beliefs or practices serve a person rather than on examining specifically what the beliefs and practices are. These models view spirituality as a multidimensional process. Regardless of one's assessment approach, spirituality is best seen as a complement to mental

Holistic Assessment

1. **Biological (medical) dimension:** What significant medical problems has the person had in the past? What problems does he or she have now? What treatment is the person receiving?
2. **Psychological dimension:** Are there any significant psychological problems? Are they being treated? If so, how?
3. **Family systems dimension:** Are there at present, or have there been in the past, patterns within the person's relationships with other family members which have contributed to or perpetuated present problems?
4. **Psychosocial dimension:** What is the history of the person's life, including place of birth and childhood home, family of origin, education, work history, and other important activities and relationships? What is the person's present living situation and what are the person's financial resources?
5. **Ethnic, racial, or cultural dimension:** What is the person's racial, ethnic, or cultural background? How does it contribute to the person's way of addressing any current concerns?
6. **Social issues dimension:** Are the present problems of the person created by or compounded by larger social problems or dysfunctions of which the person is largely a victim? If the person is in part suffering from larger social problems can he or she become aware of them and join with others in efforts to address those problems?
7. **Spiritual dimension**

Spiritual Assessment

1. **Belief and meaning:** What beliefs does the person have which give meaning and purpose to his or her life? What major symbols reflect or express meaning for this person? What is the person's story? Are there any current problems which have a specific meaning or alter established meaning? Is the person presently or has he or she in the past been affiliated with a formal system of belief (i.e., church)?
2. **Vocation and obligations:** Do the person's beliefs and sense of meanings in life create a sense of duty, vocation, calling, or moral obligation? Will any current problems cause conflict or compromise in this person's perception of his or her ability to fulfill these duties? Are any current problems viewed as a sacrifice or atonement or otherwise essential to this person's sense of duty?
3. **Experience and emotion:** What direct contacts with the sacred or divine or with the demonic has the person had? What emotions or moods are predominately associated with these contacts and with the person's beliefs, sense of meaning in life, and associated sense of vocation?
4. **Courage and growth:** Must the meaning of new experience, including any current problems, be fit into existing beliefs and symbols? Can the person let go of existing beliefs and symbols in order to allow new ones to emerge?
5. **Ritual and practice:** What are the rituals and practices associated with the person's beliefs and meaning in life? Will current problems, if any, cause a change in the rituals or practices the persons feels are required or in the person's ability to perform or participate in those which are important to him or her?
6. **Community:** Is the person part of one or more formal or informal communities of shared belief, meaning in life, ritual or practice? What is the style of the person's participation in these communities?
7. **Authority and guidance:** Where does the person find the authority for his or her beliefs, meaning in life, vocation, rituals, and practices? When faced with doubt, confusion, tragedy, or conflict, where does he or she look for guidance? To what extent does the person look outside or inside him- or herself for guidance?

FIGURE 4.5. Fitchett's 7 × 7 model for spiritual assessment. Adapted from Fitchett (1993). Copyright 1993 by Journal of Pastoral Care Publications. Adapted by permission.

health assessment. It "does not displace the accumulated empirical knowledge of mental functioning and mental health treatment" (Bergin, 1991, p. 399).

Assessing the Couple and Family System

One of the things that distinguishes family therapy is the importance it places on assessing the couple or family system in order to place the individual in proper context. Obviously, the theoretical lens that you use will influence your assessment approach with couples and families. A structural family therapist may see enmeshment or diffuse boundaries, whereas a Bowenian therapist may see fusion or an undifferentiated ego mass within the same family. However, they each tap into an underlying concept of closeness or distance. Thus, our approach in this section is to outline important areas of assessment to consider regardless of which theoretical orientation you choose. The specific way in which these issues are explored will depend on your personal style as well as your theoretical orientation.

Family Structure

The first step in the family assessment process is to obtain the family structure. If you are interested in multigenerational issues, the family structure assessment ideally should include at least three generations (e.g., child, parent, and grandparents). A genogram (McGoldrick, Gerson, & Petri, 2008) is a convenient way to capture the family structure visually. The family structure should reflect all the individuals who are significant in the client's life either by their presence or absence. For example, the family structure should include both biological parents even if the client has little or no contact with one of them, because the absence of a parent is often a therapeutic issue. Likewise, the family structure should not be restricted to biologically related relatives since other people, such as stepparents and live-in nannies, can have a significant influence on a client's life. Asking about multiple marriages and who lives with whom is often helpful in uncovering significant individuals who may not be biologically related.

The family structure can be an important source of clinical hypotheses. You could explore possible loyalty conflicts that may exist in a remarried family constellation, or discuss how a single parent without proper social support may be overwhelmed with parenting responsibilities. Likewise, hypotheses could also be generated based on the sibling constellation (birth order, gender, age difference of siblings). For example, a firstborn child may be more likely to be parentified.

Life Cycle Issues

You should also consider life cycle issues when conducting an assessment. Is the family dealing with particular life transitions, such as birth of the first child or launching children? Is the family having difficulty with these transitions? Conflict between a parent and an adolescent may be related to the adolescent seeking greater autonomy. Or is a child's need for attention being ignored as a result of a parent focusing on a new marriage? You should also consider if the life transitions are occurring in the normative range, as well as the possible presence of stressors due to life cycle issues. For example, a couple may be feeling overwhelmed by the caretaking demands of both their own children and elderly parents.

The Couple's Relationship

Assessing the couple's relationship is obviously important when doing marital or couple therapy. However, it is important for you to assess the couple relationship even if the presenting problem centers on a child. Marital or couple conflict can have a significant impact on children. For example, a parent may inappropriately turn to a child to get his or her emotional needs met if the couple relationship is not fulfilling, or a child may act out because he or she is triangulated in the parents' conflict.

A good place to start when doing a couple assessment is to administer a measure of marital adjustment or marital quality, such as the Dyadic Adjustment Scale (Spanier, 1976), the Marital Adjustment Test (Locke & Wallace, 1959), or the Marital Satisfaction Inventory (Snyder, 1979). These instruments will give you an idea of the overall level of distress in the relationship. In addition, they will quickly help you assess the areas in which the couple is having conflict (e.g., sex, finances, in-laws) or, conversely, the areas in which the couple is doing well.

You should also assess for possible issues of commitment. If the couple is not married, is one or both of the individuals ambivalent about continuing the relationship? If the couple is married, has either one seriously considered divorce? Brief pencil-and-paper instruments such as the Marital Instability Index (Edwards, Johnson, & Booth, 1987) or the Marital Status Inventory (Crane, Newfield, & Armstrong, 1984; Weiss & Cerrato, 1980) can be used to measure the likelihood the couple will divorce. You should also assess whether one or both individuals may be significantly involved with other people or activities that impact their commitment to a relationship. Is one individual having an affair? Do one or both partners spend a significant amount of time with friends, parents, or children at the expense of time with the partner? Likewise, does the amount of time that one or both partners spend at work or with hobbies negatively impact the relationship?

Assessing how issues of control and responsibility are handled in the relationship is also important. An excellent way to assess this is to explore how the couple makes decisions. Do they share decisions together, or does one person usually make the decision? Is physical violence or the threat of it used for control (see previous section on issues of harm)? Gender roles can also impact how a couple shares control and responsibility. Does the couple follow a traditional or an egalitarian model? Does the couple agree upon their roles and responsibilities within the relationship? In terms of responsibilities, does one partner overfunction while the other underfunctions?

The nature of the couple's interactions can also reveal much about their relationship bond. Does the couple do activities together, or do they lead independent lives? What types of activities (e.g., leisure, vacations, projects, church attendance, volunteer work) do they share? To what extent is the couple verbally or physically affectionate with one another? Does the couple have a satisfactory sexual relationship? If not, what is the nature of the concerns? Exploring the couple's courtship can be helpful in assessing relationship bonds. For example, what first attracted them to one another? In some cases, reviewing the courtship history may uncover that a couple has not properly bonded (e.g., deciding to marry to legitimize an unexpected pregnancy).

You should also assess a couple's communication and conflict resolution skills. In terms of communication, can the couple listen to one another? Can the couple express their thoughts and feelings to one another? In addition, are they able to take responsibility for their own feelings and actions, or do they frequently take a blaming stance? Having the couple discuss an issue while you observe their interaction can be an excellent approach to assessing communication skills. In addition, you will want to assess how the couple handles conflict. Do both partners avoid conflict, creating a conflict-avoidant pattern? Does the couple follow a demand–withdraw pattern where one individual pursues discussion of issues while the other is avoidant? Or, do both attack, resulting in conflict that can quickly escalate? If the latter, does the couple ever get physically violent during fights (see issues of harm)? Fights or conflicts often follow a predictable sequence or pattern. Identifying and interrupting this cycle or sequence can be critical to success in couple therapy. Circular questioning (see Chapter 6) can be a particularly effective tool for uncovering the pattern in a couple's fights.

You will also want to explore how the couple's relationship is impacted by children (or the lack of them). If the couple does not have children, do they plan to have children? Are there any factors (e.g., infertility, one partner does not want children) that are keeping them from having children at this time? If the couple has children, are they able to support one another or is parenting a source of conflict? Even if the couple is no longer married, you should assess the impact of children on the relationship. For example, are the parents engaged in a custody battle, or have they been able to work out an effective coparenting relationship?

Family Assessment

Like couples, families should also be assessed for issues of commitment, control, responsibility, relationship bonds, communication, and conflict resolution skills.

In terms of commitment, you should assess how committed the parent or parents are to their children. In an intact family, are both parents equally invested in parenting? In divorced or separated families, are both parents still involved with the children? If not, why? How has the child or children made sense of this? Do the parents have favorites or certain children with whom they are more invested than others? Is there a child who is a scapegoat for family problems and is being forced out of the family? It is also important to explore if one or both parents have other commitments or problems that negatively impact their parenting. For example, are the children's needs being ignored as a parent focuses energy on a new relationship or marriage? Are one or both parents focusing too much energy on work at the expense of their children? Is a mental illness or some other stressor reducing the parent's energy for managing and nurturing children?

You should also assess for possible issues of control and responsibility within the family. Consider how the parents monitor their children's activities and behavior. Assess how discipline is handled. Are the consequences for misbehavior appropriate and administered in a calm and nonreactive manner, or is there evidence of physical abuse (see previous section under issues of harm)? Are the parents consistent in enforcing the rules? You should assess if the children have developmentally appropriate levels of responsibility and privileges. Look at the responsibilities each child has. Is a child being parentified? That is, is a child knowledgeable or concerned about issues that would only be appropriate for adults? To what extent are children given age-appropriate input into making decisions?

A third important area to explore is the nature of relationship bonds between family members. Are any parent–child dyads particularly conflictual? Do the parents spend an appropriate amount of time with their children, helping with homework, playing, or taking part in other activities? Do the children receive praise from their parents, as well as verbal and physical affection? Or is the relationship primarily characterized by negativity? Do the parents rely too much on their children for their own emotional needs? Is there any evidence of sexual abuse (see issues of harm)?

When exploring the relationship bonds between family members, it is important that you consider other relationships within the family besides those of parent and child. Sibling relationships can be an important source of support for children. In addition, sibling conflict may indicate that the children are aligned with different parents, who in turn are in conflict with one another. Therefore, you should also assess what types of interactions the children have with one another. Do they do a lot of activities together? Are the relationships generally harmonious or highly conflictual? In multigenerational households, you should also assess the relationships between various family members. For example, does the child have a close or distant relationship with a grandparent who also lives in the household?

Finally, you should observe how family members communicate and resolve conflicts with one another. Are family members able to speak without being interrupted? Do family members speak for one another? Are children comfortable sharing their thoughts, feelings, or fears with their parents? Do family members have difficulty talking about certain topics or issues? Likewise, are certain emotions such as anger or sadness unacceptable to have or to express? Are family members respectful when talking to one another, or are they verbally abusive? Does conflict ever escalate to the point of one or more family members being physically aggressive with each other (see issues of harm)? Do the conflicts seem to follow a repetitive pattern?

Assessing Social Systems Outside the Family

Although as a family therapist you will be primarily concerned with assessing the couple or family system, it is important to recognize that a thorough assessment will also extend beyond these boundaries. Family members interact with a variety of social systems outside the immediate family. For example, the extended family often plays a critical role in the immediate family's life. However, schools, work, friendship networks, and neighborhoods are also important social systems to assess. In some cases, the courts, social service agencies, health and medical services, or other psychotherapists may be involved with one or more family members. A thorough assessment will consider the potential influence that each of these systems may have on the clients.

Assessing these systems outside the immediate family should be carried out with several purposes in mind. First, you should assess if stressors outside the family are contributing to the issues within the family. Stressors from work could be contributing to a couple's difficulties. Likewise, illness or other problems in the extended family could be impacting a family or couple.

Second, you should assess the degree to which individuals or systems outside the family can provide support or resources. Extended family members may be able to provide important emotional or instrumental support. Friends may also be able to provide needed help. If you find that your clients have limited support outside the family, then you may want to work with them to develop a better social support network.

Third, it is important that you assess each family member's level of functioning outside the family. Do family difficulties impact the individual's work performance? Does a child's misbehavior occur primarily at home, or is it present at school as well? Asking questions such as these will help you assess the severity of the problem. In some cases, you may find that a family member has a significantly higher level of functioning in another system—for example, a child may manifest fewer problems at school than at home. In these cases, you can take a solution-focused approach and identify what factors contribute to your client's functioning or well-being in one setting.

Fourth, assessing external systems may provide important clues to individual and interpersonal dynamics within the family. In many cases, individuals relate to people outside the family in ways similar to how they relate to family members. One client openly discussed his distrust of friends and work colleagues, which in turn illuminated his pattern of interaction with his divorced wife. Carefully assessing family members' interactions with people outside the family can uncover or validate dynamics within the family.

Finally, you should assess the potential impact that systems outside the family can have on the therapy process. Some clients, for example, are mandated to come to therapy by the courts. You will want to be clear on what the courts want to see accomplished, and what the consequences are for noncompliance. In other cases, multiple therapists might be involved with various family members. Ideally, therapists will work closely with one another to avoid working at cross-purposes.

Whenever you must work with another individual or system outside the family, the potential always exists for triangles or alliances that may interfere with the therapy process. A couple involved in divorce and a custody battle may each have their own therapist, both of whom need to be careful not to become so strongly aligned with their own client that they simply create a conflictual relationship that mirrors the conflict between the couple. In another case, you may need to guard against being triangulated between a school and family over a child's behavior.

Assessing Families within the Larger Social Context

Family therapy has been criticized in the past for ignoring the important influence that historical, social, and economic contexts have on individuals and families (Goldner, 1985; James & McIntyre, 1983; Taggart, 1985). Feminist family therapists, for example, have discussed how gender socialization and inequity in society have important implications for how men and women experience family. Just as individually oriented therapists have been said to ignore the family context of a child's misbehavior, family therapists have been accused of ignoring the societal context of family dynamics.

Gender socialization is an important contextual system that should be included in assessment. It is not uncommon for differences in gender socialization to contribute to conflicts between men and women in intimate relationships. In one case, a husband complained that his wife was always checking up on him, which he resented and saw as controlling. The wife insisted that she was simply interested in hearing how his day went and wasn't checking up on him. She felt distressed over how he angrily withdrew, which resulted in her feeling isolated and alone. This in turn increased her need for connection with her husband. For this couple, gender socialization was contributing to their cycle of distancing and pursuing. Like many men, the husband was socialized to value independence and to be sensitive to issues of status, hierarchy, and control. As a result, he interpreted her "checking in" as "checking up" on him. The couple was able to interrupt the distance–pursuit pattern through a better understanding of how gender socialization was contributing to it.

As with any generalization, however, the therapist needs to recognize that exceptions occur with regard to common gender patterns. Some women may have stereotypical male behaviors or beliefs, while some men may have stereotypical female behaviors or beliefs. Gender patterns should be regarded as hypotheses that need to be confirmed or ruled out with further assessment, not rigidly applied to all male–female dynamics.

When gender socialization is a contributing factor to a problematic dynamic, the therapist will frequently find other factors that reinforce it. For example, the dynamics of an enmeshed family of origin may reinforce the societal message that a woman receives—to take care of others' needs at the expense of her own. In the preceding case example, the husband's fear of control was reinforced by having had a controlling parent. Therefore, you should be aware that factors in addition to gender socialization may reinforce a problematic dynamic.

The racial or ethnic background of a family is also important to consider when doing assessment, particularly if it differs from your own. Sensitivity to culture is critical, beginning with the initial interview, so that a solid therapeutic relationship develops and the client remains engaged in therapy. Fortunately, respectful and sensitive awareness can instill more confidence in the therapeutic relationship. For example, one of the authors, a 115-pound, middle-class, non-drug-using Caucasian, recalls her first client in her first internship: a 250-pound, tattoo-bearing, heroin-addicted, economically disadvantaged Hispanic male. What developed was a wonderful working relationship, due to the client's willingness to educate the therapist and the therapist's ability to find empathic connections with the client.

Three general guidelines apply to a culturally sensitive assessment. First, you should consider a client's cultural background when interpreting the information gained through assessment. Therapists may misinterpret certain behaviors if they do not place them in the proper cultural context. In American culture, a child who fails to make eye contact with adults might be perceived to have poor self-esteem. However, in other cultures a child who makes direct eye contact with an adult would be showing disrespect. Likewise, be aware of your own cultural filter, because this will affect how you perceive different clients and their actions. For example, you and your clients may have different expectations regarding appropriate family communication or the way to raise children due to your different cultural backgrounds.

Second, you should not assume that group norms for specific cultural groups will automatically apply to an individual from that group. Therefore, any assumptions about an individual's behavior based on cultural norms must be regarded as tentative until they can be confirmed through further assessment. Children from a family of recent immigrants, for example, may be more acculturated to American culture than their parents or grandparents. To some degree, each family must be taken as a "case study," since the degree to which a family accepts or displays a cultural prescription is unique to that family.

Third, you should be aware of how cultural differences may influence the therapist–client relationship, and the implications that this might have for assessment. For example, members of a minority group might be reluctant to discuss sensitive information because they fear prejudice from the majority group (Garbarino & Stott, 1989). This in turn can affect a therapist's approach to assessment. Expectations for how therapy can help also need to be explored. Many cultures expect therapists to take on an authoritative role, while others expect more mutuality.

The preceding guidelines for sensitive, cross-cultural assessment can also be applied when exploring cultures that are defined by a characteristic other than race or ethnicity. Cultural differences, for example, can be anticipated between individuals who belong to different religious backgrounds, sexual orientations, social classes, and so forth. Each of these social groups has the potential to influence an individual's sense of identity, beliefs, and manner of relating to others. Therefore, you should determine which of these potential cultures is most salient to each family member and assess for its impact on the family.

However broadly one chooses to define "culture," we need to be reminded that when a family's cultural heritage is positively accessed, a clinician acquires one further resource for change. As Minuchin and Fishman (1981) point out, "Every family has elements in their own culture which, if understood and utilized, can become levers to actualize and expand the family members' behavioral repertoire" (p. 262).

CONCLUSION

In many ways, conducting a thorough assessment is a little like putting a puzzle together. The initial assessment involves putting the corner and edge pieces together first in order to get oriented to the case. Then, you begin to put the rest of the puzzle together piece by piece until a clinical picture emerges. Important pieces of the clinical puzzle include assessing for potential issues of harm, possible substance abuse concerns, and possible biological factors. You must connect these concerns to other pieces of the puzzle, such as possible psychopathology, the clients' meaning system, and issues of spirituality. These pieces in turn must interlock with social systems including couple and family relationships, relationships outside the family, and larger social systems, such as culture and gender socialization. If you address each of these interconnected pieces of the puzzle, we believe that you will obtain a complete clinical picture of your clients.

CHAPTER 5

Developing a
Treatment Focus

Bob and Alice Jones come for marital therapy because Alice is fed up. According to her, being married to Bob is like having an extra child—not a husband. Bob has been fired from several jobs in the last few years. He can't keep up with household tasks like paying the bills on time, doing the yard work, or getting to the children's games on time. In addition, Alice is sick of Bob's explosive temper when something goes wrong. While Alice's work as a physical therapist has kept the family financially afloat, she feels exhausted, sad, and discouraged most days. Bob states that he loves Alice and can't quite understand why she is so upset. At the end of the session, Bob brings up that he is even more worried about Dan, his 13-year-old son, who is not doing well in school because he "won't focus" and spends most of his time alone in his room playing video games.

It's easy to imagine that the therapist meeting Bob and Alice for the first time may be at a loss in terms of where to start. There are so many problems and Bob and Alice don't even agree on the most important issues. In addition, the therapist might have his or her own views on the initial focus of treatment. How do you decide treatment priorities—what to treat, what to ignore, in what order of priority, and so forth?

This chapter lays out ways to develop a treatment focus using clinical reasoning. It will help you to organize the assessment information you have obtained over the first few meetings with your clients and to develop a treatment plan. The treatment plan defines the problems to be addressed in the therapy and identifies the particular interventions that will be offered to address the problems. Writing an initial treatment plan begins to formalize the treatment contract with your clients.

After a beginning family therapist learns to "breathe" (i.e., make it through the first few sessions of therapy) and begins to join and assess what is going on in the family, the question "Now what do I do?" is heard by supervisors. Clinical reasoning is the process by which you begin to conceptualize (or make sense of) the problems presented using family therapy concepts. It is a time to write down what you do know from the assessment information and to hypothesize about the potential reasons for the problems. Clinical reasoning provides direction regarding who needs to attend the therapy sessions, which interventions to use, how long the therapy might last, and whether consultation with outside professionals, such as physicians and teachers, will be necessary. All family therapists need to know how to conceptualize and articulate what they do. Developing the capacity to reason clinically is essential to becoming proficient in one's professional discipline. This chapter will help you develop this capacity.

DEVELOPING A TREATMENT PLAN

A key treatment skill for family therapists is the ability to write a thorough treatment plan that outlines your focus and what you will be doing in the therapy. Developing such a plan involves a set of logical steps, as seen in Table 5.1. The first three steps can usually be written after the first one to three meetings with a client. The discipline of writing down an assessment and treatment outline at this juncture can organize treatment significantly. Try to write one within the first three sessions with your client; some agencies' policies will require a plan after your first meeting. If you get stuck, talk through the case with a supervisor or colleague. Several of the following sections detail com-

---

TABLE 5.1. Developing a Treatment Plan

Step 1: Select a problem list.

Step 2: Understand the client's goals for change.

Step 3: Conceptualize the case, including a DSM-IV-TR diagnosis.

Step 4: Establish long-term treatment goals.

Step 5: Select treatment interventions.

Step 6: Determine length and frequency of treatment.

Step 7: Consider referrals to and/or consultation with outside resources.

---

ponents of the initial treatment plan, and a case example follows at the end of the chapter.

Step 1: Select a Problem List

Step 1 in writing an initial treatment plan involves listing problems that the client presents and the therapist uncovers during the assessment. Especially in the first session (see Chapter 3), clients express their concerns regarding specific problems they are coming to therapy to manage differently. However, when the therapist conducts a thorough assessment, other problem areas may be added. For example, a couple might state that they are having difficulty communicating and often escalate into shouting matches. As the therapist assesses when this occurs, he or she may hypothesize that alcohol is a possible contributor to their interaction.

If the list includes several family or individual problems, the therapist and the family must negotiate which problem will be handled first, second, and so on. For example, if a family is struggling with agreeing on a parenting style with their adolescent daughter as well as determining if an elderly parent should move in with them, there needs to be a discussion about which of these concerns will be the priority for treatment. At times agreement can be difficult to find. For example, one partner may want to work on the marriage while the other wants to buffer the children from a harsh divorce. Beginning therapists often assume that the treatment goals are shared by family members while they actually may be in conflict.

Writing down the agreed-upon "problem priority list" begins a formalized treatment plan and helps the therapist and the family to stay focused. For example, during the first interview with the Jones family, the therapist might jot down the following problem list:

Bob Jones

Problems with work? (Get work history.)
Problems with marriage?
Anger (Check for domestic violence.)

Alice Jones

Depressed?

Dan

Depressed?
Poor school performance? (Refer out for evaluation?)

Isolated from family? (Significant family conflict in addition to marital conflict?)

Possible ADHD? (Check Dad for ADHD also.)

Couple/Family

Financial stress

Marital conflict

Lack of marital satisfaction (Why is there a difference in husband's and wife's dissatisfaction?)

Is Dan being triangulated or is he the "symptom bearer" for this stressed family?

If the family wants to change the focus of treatment, the therapist can review the list and talk with the family about it. This step is helpful for beginning therapists since one common problem is the "complaint-of-the-week client" who shifts chaotically from topic to topic. Referring to a co-created written list will help you focus your energy. It can also help the family determine when therapy can be terminated.

Step 2: Understand the Client's Goals for Change

After prioritizing problems, it's now time to understand your clients' goals in therapy—what does each person want to see changed? Family members will often say what they want other family members to change and have a harder time articulating what they might do differently. Encourage your clients to talk about changes they can make rather than simply focusing on other family members.

Step 3: Conceptualize the Case, Including a DSM-IV-TR Diagnosis

Step 3 offers a place for the conceptualization of the case, which includes a diagnostic determination using the DSM-IV-TR multiaxial assessment. In teaching, we have found that beginning family therapists become confused by the "smorgasbord" of available theoretical interpretations used to understand presenting problems. Early family therapists often identify with one particular school of family therapy. It was common in the 1970s and 1980s for family therapists to identify themselves with a particular theoretical school, as in "I'm a structural family therapist" or "I'm Bowenian." This was the era when training programs frequently taught only one or two theories, often structural and strategic family therapy. Family therapists who trained during this era would usually treat every client they saw using their favorite theoretical orientation.

In concert with Nichols and Everett (1986), we strongly advocate for an integrative approach to conceptualization and treatment. By integrative, we mean a solid foundation in systemic thinking and the consideration of multiple systems as expressed in the biopsychosocial model, which is discussed below. Our emphasis on integration does not mean, however, that therapists must forgo the use of a specific family therapy model to treat a specific part of the system. However, we hope therapists will conceptualize from many different perspectives and then decide which ones are the best fit for the client. As you will see below, multiple perspectives can coexist.

How does the therapist build a bridge between the assessment, the prioritized list of problems, and selection of goals/interventions to help the family? Clinical reasoning helps the therapist build this bridge. He or she starts with a problem to be addressed, reviews the assessment information gleaned and then hypothesizes about why the problem exists and what interventions or research suggestions are needed to address it. The therapist must be disciplined to reflect and take time to conceptualize the case using the key resources provided by their profession in order to be effective. So what are the key conceptual resources available to a family therapist? Our focus will be on systems theory, family development, and research.

A Biopsychosocial–Systems Model

The biopsychosocial model (Engel, 1977), which was developed to emphasize the interrelatedness of biological, psychological, family, and community factors in health, provides a bird's-eye view of the family. Our use of the biopsychsocial model is guided by general systems theory (GST) (Bertalanffy, 1968). GST is the theoretical foundation of family therapy and underscores the concept of *wholeness*, or the idea that "the whole is greater than the sum of its parts." Rather than reducing entities to their parts in a reductive manner, family therapists look for patterns and processes in problem descriptions and appreciate the idea that whatever affects one part of a system affects other parts of the system. A traditional family systems view means that the family, rather than the individual, is the unit of understanding and care, no matter who comes to therapy. Even when working with individuals, family therapists understand the relational and cultural contexts, recognize that there are multiple perspectives to any problem, and appreciate that we are in a responsible relationship with all members of a family system. Treatment too can be multidimensional, given this way of making sense of the issues presented.

A biopsychosocial–systems conceptual model will allow you to map the multiple systems active in a family's life—individual system, interactional system, intergenerational system, and community system—to understand how they simultaneously affect one another (Weeks, 1989; Breen Ruddy & McDaniel, 2008). After a careful assessment, you will be able to reflect on each of the aforementioned systems and make a judgment about "hot spots," or areas of needed intervention. Our approach to considering multiple systems is influenced by several integrative family therapy models, most notably the Intersystem Model developed by Gerald Weeks (1989). Within each system, you will see the influence of many family therapy models.

Individual System (Biological/Psychological). Although family therapists have historically looked to family relationships first to understand presenting problems, we still have a responsibility to consider individual factors in our hypotheses about problems. Here are a few key questions to ask when assessing individuals in systems:

- Do any family members meet the criteria for a particular mental health diagnosis? If so, what does the evidence-based literature say about how to approach that specific diagnosis?
- Do any family members have a medical problem that is impacting the family? For example, could poorly controlled Type 2 diabetes play a role in depression and family conflict?
- Are particular family members' beliefs or assumptions (e.g., cognitive distortions) contributing to the presenting problem?
- Are the ways that family members express emotions contributing to the presenting problem? How do anger, fear, and sadness get expressed (or not expressed) in the family?

Interactional System. Within every family exists a structure or organization that includes subsystems (spousal, parent–child, sibling), boundaries (diffuse, open, closed), and a hierarchy of individuals and subsystems (Minuchin, 1974). Boundaries, which regulate closeness and distance within families, and hierarchy, which displays the power within a system, provide a context for interactional patterns and an emotional milieu within a family, often referred to as family process. Here a few questions to consider when conceptualizing the interactional system:

- Is the family too enmeshed (diffuse boundaries) or too disengaged (closed boundaries)?
- Is the hierarchy flat (equal power among family members) or incongruous (children have more power than parents)?
- Are rules and roles in the couple and family poorly defined or overly rigid?
- What relationship patterns exist? For example, are the parents focusing on the child's problem to avoid their marital discord (triangling)? Is there a pursuer–distancer pattern in the couple's relationship?

Intergenerational System. The interactional system may be best understood by examining the extended family system (Bowen, 1978). Taking a historical perspective doesn't mean looking for a cause in the past to explain the present. Rather, our emphasis is on the continuation of patterns, emotions, and behaviors over at least three generations and the quality of relationships between different generations in the present. Here are a few questions to consider with regard to the intergenerational system:

- What is each parent/spouse's role in his or her family of origin? What is each adult's level of intrapersonal and interpersonal differentiation?
- What patterns exist in the multigenerational family—triangles, emotional and/or physical cutoff, distancing, overfunctioning/ underfunctioning?
- Are there any anniversary reactions that are contributing to the current problems (e.g., loss)?
- Are there any scripts/beliefs/mantras that have been passed down through the generations?

Community System. In addition to considering the interactions within multigenerational families, it is vital to consider the interactions *between* families and social systems in the community as a potential entry point in treatment. As discussed in Chapter 4, many families are engaged in meaningful, and sometimes stressful, relationships with teachers, physicians, social workers, probation officers, and others. Community systems might also be a source of support that we encourage, either by establishing linkages that don't currently exist or strengthening linkages that do. Here are a few questions to ask about community systems:

- How do family members view the community systems currently active in their lives?
- How are community systems complicating and/or improving your client's life?
- What patterns currently exist between your client and community systems?
- What community systems could potentially improve your client's life? For example, is there a job-training site or food distribution center that can assist your client in need?

After looking at your clients' presenting problem from the multiple perspectives above, you may decide to treat one system, such as the interactional system, or create a treatment plan to work on multiple systems. For example, if the focus of therapy is to address a couple's "frequent verbal fighting," the therapist might look at how the husband's high level of anxiety and wife's alcohol use patterns (individual system), poor couple communication skills (interactional system), and the husband's conflict with his mother-in-law (intergenerational system) *all* contribute to the couple's fighting and co-influence each other. In addition to focusing on areas of pathology, therapists can also identify strengths and areas of support. In the example above, the couple may have a strong connection to their religious community (community system), which could provide guidance and resources for coping with stress.

Family Development

Families coming for therapy often lack a time perspective when presenting their concerns. Often overwhelmed and immobilized by their current challenges, they tend to magnify the present moment and ignore contextual variables that could be contributing to their stress (McGoldrick & Carter, 2003; Nichols & Everett, 1986). Like their clients, therapists can also become overly focused on the current crisis rather than broadening the time frame to understand what is going on. For example, a child's acting out at school might be related to his mother's recent remarriage.

A developmental perspective is valuable in two primary ways: first, it allows you to explore and understand dysfunctional patterns throughout the system over time, not just in the present moment; and second, it helps you identify predictable and unpredictable changes in a system's natural growth and development. Predictable changes include the movement between life cycle stages, such as the transition to adolescence. Unpredictable changes could include job loss, geographical relocation and migration, serious illness, divorce, or other factors that have a major impact on family life.

The ability to work together and accommodate these changes is central to functioning as a family. According to Nichols and Everett (1986), "some families may present themselves for therapy at the onset of the [developmental] disruption, others may not feel that there is a problem until disruptive events have accumulated and ... resulted in severe symptomatology" (p. 186). One of the benefits of thinking developmentally is that it will allow you to normalize difficulties that families present in therapy. In Chapter 7, we explore predictable and unpredictable stressors in family development.

Research

Research can be another factor that influences the way a therapist conceptualizes a case. What does the research say about the etiology of particular problems and what treatments have been found to work best? A therapist, for example, might want to use an empirically supported treatment (EST) for treating a particular problem. ESTs are treatments that have been shown to be beneficial through randomized experimental studies that also meet other rigorous research criteria. The Dissemination Subcommittee of the Committee for Science and Practice within the American Psychological Association has published a list of empirically supported treatments for a variety of problems (see *www.apa.org/divisions/div12/rev_est*). For example, parent management training, which will be described in Chapter 7, is an EST that has been shown to be beneficial for oppositional defiant disorder.

Shadish and Baldwin (2003) have argued that ESTs offer too narrow a definition of what should be considered an empirically supported treatment, and suggest that meta-analytically supported treatments (MASTs) could also be used to inform clinical work. Like ESTs, treatments included in MASTs have been evaluated through randomized trials. Through meta-analysis, results from these studies are pooled together to uncover treatments that are superior to no-treatment controls. However, some of the studies included in the meta-analyses do not have clearly specified manuals or clearly delineated populations, which would exclude them from EST consideration. As a result, the list of MASTs for marriage and family interventions (see Table 5.2) offers a larger number of options relative to ESTs, although there is a significant amount of overlap between the two.

If a treatment or theory is not listed as an EST or MAST, this does not necessarily mean that it is ineffective. A number of theories or approaches have not been subject to the necessary empirical investiga-

TABLE 5.2. Meta-Analytically Supported Treatments for Marriage and Family Interventions

Treatment constructs	Supporting meta-analyses
Family interventions	
Family behavioral therapy for alcoholism	Edwards & Steinglass (1995)
Family therapy for schizophrenia[a]	Mari & Streiner (1994); Pitschel-Walz et al. (2001)
Family therapy for drug abuse	Stanton & Shadish (1997)
Family therapy for child-identified problems[a] • Behavioral/psychoeducational/problem solving • Systemic • Humanistic • Eclectic	Montgomery (1991)
Family therapy: Behavioral	Shadish et al. (1993)
Family therapy: Systemic	Shadish et al. (1993)
Family therapy: Eclectic	Shadish et al. (1993)
Family therapy: General	Shadish et al. (1993)
Marital interventions	
Marital therapy: Behavioral[a]	Dunn (1994); Dunn & Schwebel (1995); Dutcher (2000); Shadish et al. (1993); Wilson (1989)
Marital therapy: Cognitive-behavioral	Dunn (1994); Dunn & Schwebel (1995); Dutcher (2000)
Marital therapy: Systemic	Shadish et al. (1993)
Marital therapy: Eclectic	Shadish et al. (1993); Wilson (1989)
Marital therapy: Emotionally focused therapy[a]	Johnson et al. (1999)
Marital therapy • Contracting • Communication training • Contracting plus communication training • Insight oriented[a]	Plattor (1991)
Marital therapy: General	Dunn (1994); Dunn & Schwebel (1995); Dutcher (2000); Plattor (1991); Shadish et al. (1993)
Marital enrichment interventions	Hight (2000)

Note. Reprinted from Shadish and Baldwin (2003). Copyright 2003 by the American Association for Marriage and Family Therapy. Reprinted by permission of Blackwell Publishing Ltd.

[a]These treatments also appear on the list of empirically supported therapies at *www.apa.org/divisions/div12/rev_est/index.html*, as of June 2002.

tion to qualify as an EST or MAST. One of the key advantages of using an EST or MAST, however, is that the clinician has greater confidence that the treatment will be successful since there is documented evidence for its effectiveness. Therefore, you should give serious consideration to using an EST or MAST if one is available for the presenting issues you are treating. You need to be aware, however, that it may be necessary to modify your approach to best fit the needs of your clients. For example, a therapist working on marital distress might use an EST such as behavioral marital therapy as the primary treatment approach but might also need to consider making a referral for a medical evaluation if one of the individuals is struggling with significant depression.

If you are treating an individual with mental illness or a substance abuse problem, you may also want to consider reading the practice guidelines for that particular disorder published by the American Psychiatric Association. These guidelines can be accessed through the Internet at *www.psych.org/MainMenu/PsychiatricPractice/PracticeGuidelines_1. aspx*. Although the guidelines focus primarily on medication management for the disorders, they also include information about psychosocial treatments.

Step 4: Establish Long-Term Treatment Goals

In Step 4, the therapist develops appropriate therapeutic goals. These goals articulate what the therapist believes needs to change in order for the clients to realize their goals. Clients' goals state what they want to be different (e.g., less fighting), while the therapeutic goals state how the change is to occur (e.g., interruption of vicious cycle, improved communication skills).

The therapist may offer some suggestions for therapeutic goals after he or she begins to understand the problem by learning about the clients' experience and can conceptualize the beginning direction of treatment. Therapeutic goals need to be consistent or tied to the clients' goals. At times, goals of outside persons (e.g., school teachers, case workers) tied to the case must be recognized as pertinent also.

Mutual therapeutic goals are vital for the progress of therapy. A common agenda needs to be acceptable to all family members and to the therapist—that is, everyone agrees these goals are valuable to pursue in therapy. Often, beginning therapists proceed before there is a clearly defined and shared common therapeutic goal for family therapy.

At times the clients' goals may differ from those of the therapist. An angry and frustrated father who is separated from his spouse may use therapy as evidence that he is a better parent than his wife. This may not be a goal with which the therapist can agree. Mutual goals aid in establishing a collaborative, cooperative therapeutic environment where the process of therapy involves ongoing evaluation. Once therapeutic goals have been established, the therapist and clients will evaluate their progress together. Identifying realistic goals helps us determine what can be accomplished in the course of therapy. Tangible behavioral changes, such as decreasing arguments or quitting consumption of alcohol, can be observed and quantified. Changes in attitude or personal feelings are less tangible and more difficult to measure.

Although the therapist must provide the family with hope that change can happen, it is equally important to be realistic about the limits of therapy. In a summation of some major findings on psychotherapy, Grunebaum (1988) notes that couple and family therapy is helpful for probably about two-thirds to three-quarters of all clients seen. This indicates that between 25 and 33% of clients will not benefit from therapy. Nichols (1988) describes one of the contraindications of marital therapy as a couple's refusal or inability to engage in it. For example, extreme hostility and continuous nonproductive communication may make progress in couple therapy impossible. If therapy is going to move beyond support to assist the clients in making changes, there must be some cooperation and motivation to change on the part of the family.

Factors outside therapy, such as socioeconomic issues or a lack of adequate community resources, can impact the client's ability to set treatment goals. A 27-year-old single mother of two children with a limited education, living in an inner city, must address issues of economic survival before she is able to consider her own or her family's psychological well-being. The therapist may adapt the therapeutic goals to provide support, information, and resources to this client and assist her in achieving a level of stability rather than seeking to assist her in change.

A client's history and any preexisting psychopathology must be considered in evaluating treatment goals. The family's history of previous treatment is very useful diagnostic and treatment planning information. Too often therapists do not obtain a previous history because they find it dated or irrelevant to their therapy. However, information from a previous therapist can help determine what interventions will be more effective and what might be unproductive. How the family is likely or unlikely to change may become clearer.

Step 5: Select Treatment Interventions

In Step 5, the therapist must determine how he or she will address the problems from the standpoint of family therapy goals and interventions. Your theoretical training becomes essential here. What do we offer to a family that is stuck in troubling interactions? What do we have to offer a suicidal adolescent, or a couple seeking assistance after an affair, or a child who does not want to go to school? Which family members need to be involved in the treatment? Which modality of treatment will we use—will individual, couple, family, or group therapy be more effective? Most beginning therapists and many seasoned therapists can become confused here.

Interventions can be thought of as tools in the therapist's toolbox. You need a hammer, screwdriver, nails, pliers, and so forth in order to build a room addition. It also takes time to learn how to use the tools skillfully and to know what tool works best in what situation. It is common for students to seek out and embrace one approach or one "master therapist" with the hope of decreasing complexity and locating a correct path to change. That would be like using only one tool in the toolbox. We don't recommend such an approach. We hope students will learn a wide range of family therapy concepts and their associated interventions, learn to integrate them over time, and choose interventions that emerge from the integrative conceptual map suggested in Step 3 above. We agree with Nichols and Everett (1986) that "the first field to master is family. Therapy comes second" (p. 79). In Chapter 6, we discuss core family therapy interventions from multiple perspectives in more detail.

Step 6: Determine Length and Frequency of Treatment

Step 6 estimates length of therapy and how often we will be working with the client, determining if the case is appropriate for crisis, brief, or longer-term treatment. Frequency of meetings must also be decided. In the past, most therapists and clients never made an explicit decision about the length of treatment. Treatment started and lasted as long as the clients or the therapist wanted. The therapy might have slowly evolved over time, so even when the presenting problem was resolved, therapy continued as new issues emerged. The historical influence of psychoanalysis, in which therapy was frequent and lasted over several years, probably led most people to think of therapy as at least a year-long venture.

Except for those who pay independently for mental health services, this is no longer the situation. Concerns about cost and the lack of empirical support for the contention that longer therapy is, in fact, more successful have led to a growing trend toward brief, time-limited treatments. Today, therapy may be time-limited because the payer sets a limit on the number of sessions allowed. Length of therapy is no longer a decision made by the therapist and client but is strongly influenced by other considerations.

Family therapy has always tended toward brief, problem-focused treatments. For some approaches, the average number of sessions is about six. Family therapists focus on a specific problem and when that problem is solved, the therapy ends. When tangential issues arise, they are addressed only in relation to the presenting problem. For example, a client comes in because he feels unable to form a lasting, intimate relationship. During the third session he mentions that he also feels overweight and unable to lose weight. Instead of redirecting the focus, the matter would be addressed only in terms of how it influences the client's initiatives in forming relationships.

Beginning family therapists make two common mistakes regarding the length of therapy. First, even when they have set therapeutic goals, they change the focus each session depending on the "problem of the week." In our program, we begin to identify "problem of the week" families and recognize that therapy with them may go on forever. Another common problem is that the therapist and family meet the stated goal and decide to keep doing therapy anyway. An important skill for a beginning therapist is to know when to end therapy (see Chapter 11 for a detailed discussion of termination). This criterion should be at least partially established when the goals are set. Thus, therapy ends when the goals are met, and goals are set using a realistic timetable.

While insurance companies may play a role in determining length of treatment, clearly it is the client and the nature of the problem that should guide the therapist in deciding the best modality of treatment— either crisis intervention, brief therapy, or long-term treatment. Table 5.3 provides a number of helpful indicators that can be used when making decisions about length of therapy.

Frequency of sessions may range from several times a week if the family is in severe crisis to a regular monthly appointment over a period of several months. Clients can also be seen following termination for a follow-up or checkup session. Sessions can be held with greater frequency at the beginning of therapy, weekly for example, and move to every other week as the family progresses and moves toward termination.

Frequency of sessions is determined by practical and logistical issues as well as clinical or treatment concerns. As mentioned earlier,

TABLE 5.3. Length of Therapy Indicators

Indicators for crisis intervention

1. There is a severe disruption in client's or family's normal functioning.
2. Client is extremely overwhelmed and highly stressed in response to an event.
3. A sudden external event has caused considerable psychological or emotional instability.
4. Family or client has been traumatized by an external event or a developmental change.
5. Client is in danger of harming self or others.
6. Client's symptoms have intensified to the point of causing incapacitation.

Indicators for brief therapy

1. Agency or institutional policy dictates a limited number of visits.
2. Client's goals for therapy are essentially symptom-focused.
3. Client or family is receptive to therapy and willing to change.
4. Client or family has additional resources available to support and integrate change.
5. Clear changes in behavior can be observed.
6. Client's or family's history is not a primary concern.

Indicators for long-term therapy

1. Client's or family's history has significant bearing on presenting concerns.
2. Client or family can engage in a longer-term therapeutic relationship.
3. Client's concerns go beyond behavioral issues and involve underlying dynamics or causes.
4. Client's goals for therapy include identifying and sustaining changes during therapy.
5. There is a significant amount of anxiety and concern that warrants longer-term work.

external guidelines may be imposed by an agency, a health maintenance organization, or the client's insurance company, which may set a limit on the number of sessions per week. It is common practice for therapy to be limited to a maximum of two sessions per week with no more than one session on a given day. Time, money, and scheduling factors may also affect session frequency. Coordinating client and therapist schedules can place some limits on available times. In couple and family therapy there tends to be a premium on late-afternoon appointments. Also, some clinics might contract services at both a school and an outpatient agency, that is, some appointments might be with an individual student at school, while other appointments might be with the parents and/or entire family at the agency.

The client's need and level of motivation will assist in determining the session frequency. Highly anxious clients may need to come in more frequently at first, in order to work toward their stated goals:

More frequent visits allow them to solve problems over a shorter period of time.

Sessions staggered over a longer period, perhaps every second or third week, can be used to determine how changes are being integrated. If the client is seen less frequently, then the therapy may be used to process changes that have occurred and evaluate their impact. In this context, therapy can support and pace changes that have happened between sessions. Periodic meetings can be scheduled after termination on an as-needed basis. Therapy should be viewed as a safe place to return to without the client feeling like a failure. Follow-up sessions should offer a review of progress that has occurred and support for the client's successes.

In addition to determining how often sessions should occur, therapists need to decide how long individual meetings will last. Tradition suggests sessions of 45–50 minutes, or perhaps 90 minutes for a family session. Clearly, most meetings have a beginning, middle, and an end. The therapist needs to pace the session so that the ending is not abrupt, but anticipated. Moving toward a summary with 10 or 15 minutes left to go can be helpful in providing adequate closure.

Step 7: Consider Referrals and/or Consultations

Step 7 reminds the family therapist that other professional or community involvement may enhance quality care. Medication referrals or psychological testing can maximize the care we provide. Connection with a cultural or religious community leader might have value in a given clinical case. Again, a biospsychosocial perspective will often help guide the referrals needed.

Knowing the resources available within the community is a necessary part of your responsibilities as a family therapist. This may include purchasing local directories of clinical services and resources, having some working knowledge of self-help groups, and networking with other professionals who provide expertise in specific areas. Agencies often organize this information better than private practitioners do, and it often takes 6 months to a year to have a solid handle on local resources if the community is a large one. Having access to outside resources enables therapists to provide clients with a written list of supplemental contacts they might find helpful. Clients often see this move as enhancing rather than detracting from the authority of the therapist.

Referrals to other mental health professionals also might be considered, particularly when there is limited progress in therapy or the therapist feels in over his or her head. Often it's helpful to discuss this feeling with the client, allowing the client either to provide reassurance that therapy is working, or to better clarify his or her needs. Beginning therapists think this kind of discussion will undermine their authority; our experience as supervisors indicates the opposite. Clients often appreciate the therapist's concern and begin to emphasize what is "working differently" in their relationships, which in turn helps to advance positive clinical work. One warning, however—some clients, especially those with abandonment issues, might interpret a discussion about referrals as meaning that you don't want to work with them. With these clients one needs to be particularly careful. Getting supervision will be important before bringing up this topic (see the discussion of supervisory consultations in Chapter 10).

An essential quality of a competent therapist working from a biopsychosocial perspective is acknowledgment of the limits of one's particular field of knowledge. During treatment planning especially, therapists are encouraged to consider consultations with other healthcare professionals. Generally, the success of referrals for medication or testing consultations depends on the therapist's ability to be clear and concise about what information he or she hopes to obtain from the referrals. The following sections highlight indications, procedures, and special considerations related to consultations with medical and psychological professionals.

Medication Consultations

Family therapists have been reticent about using psychotropic medications as part of their treatment planning (Patterson & Magulac, 1994). In fact, in the early years of family therapy, using medication could be seen as an admission of failure. Recently, attitudes about using medication have changed. Therapists who do not have a medical degree and thus cannot prescribe medication are becoming open to a joint treatment model wherein they work with a physician (usually a psychiatrist, internist, family physician, or pediatrician) in coordinating treatment (Patterson, Albala, McCahill, & Edwards, 2006). The physician prescribes and manages the psychotropic medication while the therapist provides the "talk therapy."

Family therapists need to make medication referrals with caution. Negative side effects of medication are common. In addition, patients can interpret the referral as the therapist saying "You are really crazy—too crazy for family therapy" or as the therapist abandoning the client to another provider. However, medication should not be overlooked as an option. Frequently, family therapists have no training or knowledge about psychotropic medications and have limited biological knowledge; thus, they do not consider medication as a possible intervention. In addition, therapists fear losing control of their client's treatment or view referral to another provider as a sign of failure or inadequacy. For all these reasons, family therapists might not consider making a medication referral.

While many family therapists support the idea of a biopsychosocial model of assessment and treatment, the biological part is rarely emphasized or even considered. However, a true biopsychosocial model would consider both assessment of biological influences, such as genetic history, and biologically based treatment, including medication and surgery. This holistic approach argues for including a biomedical provider if the therapist does not have expertise in biological assessment.

Beyond the biopsychosocial model, other factors compel therapists to consider medication consultations. One is that their clients ask about them. Research in the last 20 years has produced powerful new psychotropic medications with fewer negative side effects. Popular articles on the success of these new drugs can be found on any newsstand. Another reason therapists might consider medication is that they may work in a setting where the biomedical model is paramount and physicians are in charge. Health maintenance organizations and preferred provider organizations encourage medication use because it is often a relatively inexpensive, effective treatment.

Speed of treatment is another reason therapists consider medication. Timeliness and cost are key criteria in many therapy settings. While some may consider it sloppy treatment, many therapists feel pressure to use a shotgun approach in which every possible treatment is given to the patient. Since medication can bring rapid symptomatic improvement, there is increasing emphasis on using medication from the start of treatment (McNeil, 2001).

Changes within the profession also account for the growing awareness of medication. The early years of family therapy were characterized by a period of marking boundaries and separating from mainstream, traditional mental health treatments. As family therapy has become an established profession, magnifying these distinctions has become less important. Instead of acknowledging only the family as the patient, most family therapists today will recognize one family member as perhaps needing a biologically based treatment while the rest of the therapy remains focused on family interaction. Although family therapists cannot prescribe or monitor medications, they have an obligation to clients to assess for or otherwise recognize various problems and pathologies that might benefit from treatment with psychotropic drugs. Knowing when and how to obtain a psychiatric consultation is an important part of our work, as the following case demonstrates.

Bill, a 39-year-old man, presented with marital problems including constant arguing, financial problems, and a lack of mutual interests. Mary, his wife, was a 37-year-old woman who had just begun to work full-time as an insurance sales agent. She complained about Bill's moodiness and lack of involvement with the family, saying, "All he wants to do is to be left alone." Bill had worked as a stockbroker for the previous 10 years and indicated that business had been bad and was taking up more of his time than usual. This couple was seen in marital therapy for four visits. The husband quickly identified himself as "the problem," and said he felt an inability to control the way he felt and his negative attitude. He also expressed some anger toward his wife for her lack of support, particularly since she had started working full-time. The wife said that she felt she had been supporting her husband for years and needed to do something for herself. Both indicated that they felt lonely in their relationship and had little understanding of how things had deteriorated to this point of dissatisfaction. Further exploration of their individual issues indicated that the husband displayed several depressive symptoms, including a poor appetite, an erratic sleep pattern, a lack of energy, and irritability. He said he had been feeling "down" for the past several years and really couldn't remember when it seemed to have started. Family history indicated that he felt traumatized and partially responsible for his brother's accidental death when Bill was 14.

The duration and magnitude of Bill's depressive symptoms indicated that an evaluation for antidepressant medication was warranted. Since the marriage was presented as the primary problem, it was anticipated that either Bill or his wife might be reluctant to consider medication. They didn't come to marital therapy expecting to see a physician in addition to a couple therapist. They both had some preconceived beliefs about the uses of psychopharmacological drugs. Some discussion of their experiences with medications and education about psychotropic drugs was necessary. It was also important for the therapist to present Bill's need for a medication evaluation as being in the couple's best interest. Referrals are most effective if they are presented as beneficial to the client. In this case, Bill was receptive to seeing a psychiatrist for a medical evaluation. His wife's primary concern was that medication was "a crutch and addicting." It was suggested that she see the psychiatrist with her husband in order to find answers to any questions and concerns. Both agreed to go to the initial appointment.

Finally, family therapists cannot ignore the burgeoning research indicating a biological role for at least some mental disorders, such as schizophrenia, bipolar disorder, and other diseases thought previously to originate in dysfunctional family patterns. Recognizing a biological etiology naturally leads to a biological treatment, frequently medication.

With increasing public awareness about medication, the family therapist needs to learn more about psychotropic drugs. Perhaps one of the best ways to learn is through on-the-job training—experience is a powerful influence in demonstrating the efficacy of medication for certain problems. Establishing a professional relationship with a psychiatrist or primary care physician who is willing to use a joint treatment model is an ideal way to learn about medication. If possible, we try to personally know the physicians we are sending our patients to for medical evaluations so that we can be sure of both their competence and interpersonal skills. Other possibilities include participating in a continuing education course or reading one of the many books on psychotropic medications for nonphysicians. A brief "primer" on commonly used medications is provided in Table 5.4.

Psychological Testing Consultations

Another consultation possibility is to refer a client for psychological testing to obtain a more standardized report on observations the therapist has already made or a more in-depth description of some aspect of a client's life. When making a testing referral, the therapist should be as specific as possible about what he or she would like to learn. Therapists should be familiar with the variety of tests available and know what to ask for. Whereas one would use a physician for a medication consultation, psychologists are the mental health professionals with specialty training in tests and measures. Usually a report is written based on the tests the psychologist administers. Major types of tests include intelligence tests, projective tests, self-report instruments that describe some aspect of the client's emotional life, and behavioral checklists.

Testing is most commonly used in psychiatric hospitals, school settings, forensic work, and other institutional settings where standardized information beyond the therapist's clinical observations is sought. For example, parents and teachers may request testing when they have a concern about a child's behaviors or abilities. Legal experts may request testing when they are concerned about their client's mental stability or cognitive capacities. A typical psychological report would include the following information: reason for testing and referral source, brief history and description of the client, tests administered, test results, and recommendations.

When would a family therapist ask for psychological testing? Besides the legal and academic reasons just mentioned, the therapist might consider testing in the following situations:

TABLE 5.4. Psychotropic Drug Primer

Drugs for depression

SSRIs and SNRIs	Selective serotonin reuptake inhibitors (SSRIs) are the primary drug treatment for depression. Some major SSRIs include citalopram (Celexa), escitalopram (Lexapro), fluoxetine (Prozac), paroxetine (Paxil), and sertraline (Zoloft). Serotonin-norepinephrine reuptake inhibitors (SNRIs) such as venlafaxine (Effexor) and duloxetine (Cymbalta) appear to be equally effective. The only SSRI approved by the Food and Drug Administration for treatment of adolescents and children is fluoxetine (Prozac).
Tricyclics	Patients who do not respond to an SSRI or SNRI may benefit from a tricyclic antidepressant. Major tricyclics include imipramine (Tofranil), amitriptyline (Elavil), desipramine (Norpramin), and nortriptyline (Pamelor). Tricyclic treatment failure is often caused by inadequate dosage, insufficient duration of treatment, and poor compliance. Monitoring is critical.
MAO inhibitors	Phenelzine (Nardil) or tranylcypromine (Parnate) is used for patients who cannot tolerate or do not respond to SSRIs, SNRIs, or tricyclics. Subtypes of depression may benefit from these. Severe depression with psychotic symptoms may require antipsychotic drugs with an antidepressant.
Other drugs	Bupropion (Wellbutrin) may be an alternative for patients who cannot tolerate the negative side effects that may occur with other antidepressants. Mirtazapine (Remeron) and nefazodone (Serzone) have sedating properties that can be helpful in patients with marked insomnia or agitation. Trazodone (Desyrel) is frequently used along with an SSRI for this reason; however, its safety and effectiveness are unclear.
Nondrug therapy	Electroconvulsive therapy (ECT) has been used for depression that is resistant to antidepressants and may be superior for severely depressed patients, those with delusions or psychomotor retardation, suicidal patients, and some elderly patients. Vagus nerve stimulation (VNS) has also been approved for drug-resistant depression, but its effectiveness is not clear.
Adverse effects	*SSRIs and SNRIs:* jitteriness and insomnia early in treatment, nausea, diarrhea, headache, fatigue, sexual dysfunction (anorgasmia). Weight gain can occur with continued use. Serotonin syndrome is rare (most often caused by interaction with an MAO inhibitor) but is potentially fatal. Symptoms include altered mental status, fever, tachycardia, tremor, hypertension, ataxia, and gastrointestinal symptoms. *Tricyclics:* anticholinergic effects, orthostatic hypotension, sedation, weight gain, withdrawal symptoms. Overdosage can be lethal (reactions include cardiac arrhythmias, hypotension, convulsions, and coma). *MAO inhibitors:* hypertensive reactions, sexual dysfunction, weight gain, potentially fatal interactions with some other drugs and certain foods.

Note: Treatment of bipolar depression with an antidepressant alone may trigger a manic episode. Bipolar disorder is usually treated with lithium; if depression develops, an antidepressant may be added.

(cont.)

TABLE 5.4. *(cont.)*

Drugs for anxiety

Benzodiazepines	Includes diazepam (Valium), alprazolam (Xanax), lorazepam (Ativan), oxazepam (Serax), and clonazepam (Klonopin). Benzodiazepines have a high risk of pharmacological dependence and should be limited to short-term or intermittent use. "Alprazolam may cause rebound anxiety between doses and has been associated with a withdrawal syndrome, including seizures" (p. 40).
Buspirone	BuSpar, a nonbenzodiazepine antianxiety drug, does not cause sedation or functional impairment, or have high potential for abuse. Takes 1–2 weeks for results.
Propranolol	Inderal and other beta-blockers are useful in preventing performance anxiety or "stage fright" by suppressing peripheral autonomic symptoms of anxiety.
Antidepressants	Some antidepressants may be used for symptom relief of anxiety disorders. Clomipramine (Anafranil), fluvoxamine (Luvox), fluoxetine (Prozac), sertraline (Zoloft), and paroxetine (Paxil) are the drugs of choice for obsessive-compulsive disorder. For highly anxious patients with obsessive-compulsive disorder, adding a benzodiazepine or antipsychotic drug may be beneficial. SSRIs and MAO inhibitors including paroxetine (Paxil), sertraline (Zoloft), and venlafaxine (Effexor), are the most effective treatments for social anxiety disorder. Posttraumatic stress disorder is most frequently treated with an SSRI; however, MAO inhibitors and tricyclics may also be beneficial.
Adverse effects	*Benzodiazepines:* undesirable degree of sedation, anterograde amnesia, dependence (with chronic use), withdrawal (gradual tapering is important), rebound anxiety. Potentially dangerous if taken with other central nervous system depressants (e.g., alcohol, barbiturates). Some risks have been associated with use during pregnancy; however, the results are controversial. *Buspirone:* headache, dizziness, nausea, and nervousness. *Fluvoxamine:* same adverse effects as other SSRIs but with a significant number of potential drug interactions.

Drugs for bipolar disorder

Lithium	Lithium (Eskalith and others) is used for long-term maintenance to prevent depressive and manic episodes in bipolar disorder. Because lithium takes 2–3 weeks to have an effect, acutely manic patients may be treated temporarily with antipsychotic drugs such as chlorpromazine (Thorazine) or haloperidol (Haldol). During depressive episodes, a tricyclic or MAO inhibitor may be used in addition to lithium.
Other drugs	Anticonvulsant drugs including valproate (Depakote), carbamazepine (Tegretol), and lamotrigine (Lamictal) are frequently used in place of lithium. Atypical (second-generation) antipsychotic drugs such as aripiprazole (Abilify), risperidone (Risperdal), ziprasidone (Geodon), olanzapine (Symbyax, Zyprexa), and quetiapine (Seroquel) can be used.
Adverse effects	*Lithium:* nausea and fatigue in first weeks of treatment; tremor, thirst, polyuria, edema, weight gain may persist throughout treatment; confusion and ataxia are toxic effects that may not be perceived as drug induced; skin reactions (acne, psoriasis); thyroid disturbances (primarily hypothyroidism), which can exacerbate bipolar symptoms; cardiac and

(cont.)

TABLE 5.4. *(cont.)*

other birth defects. Patients on lithium should avoid pregnancy and should not breastfeed infants. *Valproate:* sedation, weight gain, nausea, diarrhea, and tremor. Fatal hepatoxicity and polycystic ovary syndrome have occurred rarely. *Carbamazepine:* rash, dizziness, diplopia, nausea, somnolence, headache, hypotremia, and many adverse drug reactions. *Lamotrigine:* nausea, dizziness, and somnolence. *Atypical antipsychotics:* somnolence, diabetes mellitus, dyslipidemia. Weight gain and diabetes mellitus are particularly common with olanzapine.

<u>Drugs for obsessive-compulsive disorder</u>

Included under "Drugs for anxiety."

<u>Drugs for psychotic disorders</u>

Atypical (second generation)	Atypical (second-generation) antipsychotics are now more widely used than first-generation, conventional antipsychotics. Although efficacy advantages have not (except for clozapine) been unequivocally demonstrated, they are better tolerated and have less serious side effects. Clozapine (Clozaril) is effective in patients with schizophrenia who are resistant to other treatment and better reduces the risk of suicide than first-generation antipsychotics. Other atypical antipsychotics include aripiprazole (Abilify), olanzapine (Zyprexa), quetiapine (Seroquel), risperidone (Risperdal), and ziprasidone (Geodon).
First generation	Conventional antipsychotic drugs include such medications as chlorpromazine (Thorazine), fluphenazine (Prolixin), perphenazine (Trilafon), haloperidol (Haldol), thioridazine (Mellaril), thiothixene (Navane), and trifluoperazine (Stelazine). Symptoms of acute psychosis may improve rapidly after treatment with antipsychotic drugs, but chronic schizophrenia requires 3 or more weeks before a benefit is seen and full improvement may take months. Many chronic patients require prolonged maintenance therapy, but the benefits may be limited and the risk of tardive dyskinesia is considerable.
Adverse effects	*First generation:* anticholinergic effects (dry mouth, constipation, etc.), drowsiness, postural hypotension, extrapyramidal effects (rigidity, akinesia, tremor), tardive dyskinesia (involuntary movements of lips, tongue, fingers, toes, or trunk), sexual dysfunction, hyperprolactinemia, and neuroleptic malignant syndrome. *Second generation:* hyperglycemia, diabetes, and weight gain. Other possible side effects include hyperlipidemia, postural hypotension, insomnia, constipation, somnolence, akathesia, anxiety, and headache. Less likely to cause extrapyramidal effects, tardive dykinesia, and neuroleptic malignant syndrome than first-generation antipsychotics. Increased risk of death among elderly patients with dementia (similar effects are seen with first-generation antipsychotics as well).

Note. Adapted from "Drugs for Psychiatric Disorders" (2006). Copyright 2006 by *The Medical Letter.* Adapted by permission.

1. A client is not processing information or following the conversation (e.g., signs of possible cognitive problems).
2. The client displays aberrant, inappropriate behavior.
3. A mental status exam reveals problems.
4. A client shows signs of a major mental disorder.
5. Corroborative information is needed for legal purposes.
6. A student is referred to therapy for learning, emotional, and/or behavioral problems.

There are also reasons not to do testing. Clients can experience psychological testing as intrusive and tedious, or they may see little reason to participate. Referral to a consultant also brings in another professional and an additional therapeutic relationship. The therapist or the client may be concerned about privacy and confidentiality, and want as little formal documentation as possible. Psychological testing can be expensive, and clients or third-party payers may be reluctant to bear the added expense.

If testing is done, the family therapist, the clients, and the recommending agency frequently find the results to be helpful, but this is not always the case. Family therapists need basic tools to evaluate the quality of the report. Probably the most common criticism of test results is that they are too vague or abstract. Having read the results, the therapist might respond, "So what?" The report will have value when it offers information pertinent to the direction of treatment.

To improve the chances of receiving a relevant report, a family therapist can become familiar with what tests are available and the qualities of a good report. One way to identify a helpful test is to take some (e.g., the Minnesota Multiphasic Personality Inventory [MMPI] or a family therapy instrument like the Dyadic Adjustment Scale) and consider whether the information is useful. Another helpful thing to do is to read a number of testing reports; quality reports will stand out. Family therapists frequently learn about two or three psychologists in their community who do excellent evaluations of children, adults, or specific areas such as memory. Asking these examiners to do evaluations of some of the therapist's own clients will begin the collaborative relationship.

A SAMPLE TREATMENT PLAN

Kelly, a Caucasian woman in her mid-50s, came to a medical clinic with a variety of health concerns, including a foot fracture and grief related to the death of her husband 8 months earlier from leukemia (see Figure

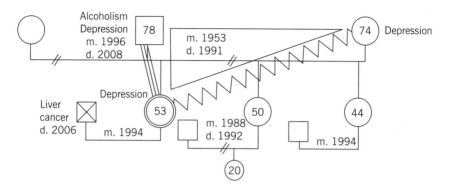

FIGURE 5.1. Genogram.

5.1). She was referred to a family therapist to help her cope with grief
and the many complicating factors that accompanied her grief. Kelly
was new to San Diego: She had lived in Philadelphia for most of her
life and moved to San Diego with her husband 5 months prior to his
death in order to be closer to her mother and two sisters. After her husband's death, Kelly did not have any income, her savings were almost
completely depleted, and she had no health insurance. Her younger
sister provided time-limited financial assistance with the expectation
that Kelly would eventually secure a job to pay for her living expenses.
At a time when Kelly wanted to fully experience and work through her
grief, she was forced to seek employment that would both cover her
expenses and not overburden her with stress. Making matters worse,
Kelly had long-standing conflictual relationships with her mother and
her youngest sister; she perceived them as uncaring and unsupportive,
which exacerbated her sense of loneliness and isolation and further
complicated her grief process.

Step 1: Select a Problem List

1. Complicated grief associated with death of husband.
2. Unemployment accompanied by a lack of financial resources.
3. Conflict with mother and younger sister.
4. Lack of support network due to living in new city.

Step 2: Understand the Client's Goals for Change

1. Cope with grief associated with loss of spouse.
2. Secure employment to pay for basic living expenses.
3. Increase skills to cope with stress.

Step 3: Conceptualize the Case, Including a DSM-IV-TR Diagnosis

Kelly is the oldest of three daughters from a chaotically enmeshed family system. She was triangulated by her parents throughout their conflictual marriage and divorce, often serving as a support to her father, who suffered from major depression and alcoholism and attempted suicide on two occasions. The coalition with her father created tension between Kelly, her mother, and her sisters. Diffuse boundaries in relationships and family conflict have been consistent themes in her life. For example, Kelly had multiple sexual affairs with men during her marriage, which has contributed to feelings of guilt in her grief.

> Axis I—Major depressive disorder, recurrent (DSM-IV-TR 296.32).
> Axis II—Obsessive-compulsive personality disorder (DSM-IV-TR 301.4).
> Axis III—None.
> Axis IV—Death of spouse; inadequate social support; inadequate finances; relational problem.

Step 4: Establish Long-Term Treatment Goals

1. Address blocks to natural grief: (a) Help client understand the complicated nature of grief; (b) help client continue life with the pleasant memories of her husband; and (c) help client engage in a rewarding life without her husband (Shear, Frank, Houck, & Reynolds, 2005).
2. Identify community resources to assist Kelly in preparing for and locating employment opportunities.
3. Improve conflict management in her relationships with mother and sister.
4. Strengthen Kelly's support network and help her define appropriate boundaries in relationships.
5. Collaborate with Kelly's primary care physician.

Step 5: Choose Treatment Interventions

1. Individual therapy to address complicated grief: Revisiting of the death; imagined conversations with her deceased husband; reengage with memories; revisit satisfying activities and places that are currently avoided.
2. Invite mother and younger sister to sessions to elicit perspec-

tives, open communication, and bring to light the private realities of each family member.

3. Talk with Kelly's primary care provider about a referral to a psychiatrist for a medication evaluation.

Step 6: Determine Length and Frequency of Treatment

Twelve to 15 sessions; weekly.

Step 7: Consider Referrals to and/or Consultation with Outside Resources

1. In collaboration with primary care provider, refer for a medication evaluation with a psychiatrist at free clinic.
2. Refer Kelly to support group for grieving spouses at local hospice.

VARIABLES THAT IMPACT TREATMENT

Financial Constraints

If your client holds insurance that pays for two to three sessions at 80%, then pays 50% for another six sessions, then nothing, he or she may want to use a "quicker fix" orientation due to these financial concerns. You may feel pressured to use a brief therapy model that focuses on a specific problem with the goal of reducing or eliminating the client's distress. Underlying issues that may contribute to the cause of the problem, such as family of origin conflicts, may not be adequately addressed within this brief therapy framework. The therapist can negotiate whether the client wishes to pay for services beyond what is provided by insurance benefits. Clearly, the role of the healthcare system in limiting the type and length of mental health services continues to shape our field. Therapists must be able to offer clinically reasonable treatment plans as they become more accountable to the payers of their clients' benefits.

Client's Availability and Motivation

Practical considerations often play a significant role. One or more persons in the family may not be available or willing to take part in treatment on a regular basis. Also, it is often difficult for clients to attend therapy between 9:00 and 5:00 on weekdays.

The therapist might also offer different options to clients regarding the way therapy will be conducted. This is especially helpful for a family that has been in therapy before. Recently, a couple came in for help with their 11-year-old daughter and reported that they had been in therapy of some sort for about 7 years of this child's life. What had already been tried, and had worked or failed, needed to be determined and discussed before moving into the treatment focus. The parents stated that they had already looked at their own childhoods. They thought that certain behavioral strategies were helpful, but they needed to adapt them to the needs of an older child. They also found themselves at odds with each other, and knew they needed help in working together on their discipline.

CONCLUSION

Developing a treatment focus allows the beginning therapist to move from being a good listener to becoming a professional. By using an initial treatment plan, you will be able to conceptualize and explain how therapy will address the painful presenting problems brought to you. Suggestions on who needs to be in therapy, how long the therapy may last, and what methods you will use can be articulated and offered to the family. Networking with other professionals or community groups may also benefit clinical care.

The family therapist balances the relational, therapeutic, and ethical concerns of practice. It is a taxing role, yet very rewarding. Creativity and professional knowledge combine to help persons in the healing process. The basic treatment skills discussed must be coordinated with the art of matching these skills to particular clients with particular problems, keeping in mind the kind of therapist you are. This is a lifelong and challenging component of being a family therapist.

CHAPTER 6

Basic Treatment Skills and Interventions

Karen and Rick stare at each other in frustration. Karen begins, "You don't help with the kids. I can't even ... " Rick interrupts, "You're too sensitive. What about the time I took the kids all afternoon ... ?" Karen rolls her eyes. Sammy, age 9, interrupts, "Don't yell. I can't stand it when you yell." There is an awkward silence in the therapy room.

What skills are necessary to be an effective therapist with a family like this? In this chapter, we first review the elements crucial to relating to your clients. Effective therapists display common qualities no matter what theory or intervention they use. Next, we discuss some basic counseling skills that are the foundation of solid therapeutic work. Finally, marriage and family therapists hold a unique repertoire of skills related to their systems perspective. These skills need to be selected intentionally, and several guidelines will be offered emphasizing the therapist's role and responsibility in this selection.

THE RUSH TO INTERVENTION
VERSUS DEVELOPING A RELATIONSHIP

Research on the effectiveness of therapy has identified one variable as critical in predicting a positive outcome. While therapists focus on compelling theoretical models or powerful techniques, research suggests that the therapist–client relationship is the most important variable, and, more specifically, the client's perception of the therapist and the relationship (Baldwin, Wampold, & Imel, 2007; Grunebaum, 1988; Miller, Duncan, & Hubble, 1997). Acknowledging the powerful impact of the therapeutic relationship is both a sobering and humbling experience.

Beginning family therapists who are overwhelmed by their clients' problems and their own sense of inadequacy are often impatient to "do something" in the therapy session. Family therapy students are especially vulnerable to the "do-something syndrome" because their training has usually involved watching numerous master therapists perform brilliant therapeutic techniques on videos. After watching several of these videos and hearing about the success of their classmates, students are left wondering why nothing dramatic is happening in their sessions, and the pressure for something to happen intensifies.

This "do-something syndrome" is unfortunate because students fail to recognize their most powerful therapeutic tool—themselves. Often in supervision, we suggest that students sit back, relax, and simply try to get to know and understand the client and his or her story. The point is that before technique and theory can be effective, there must be a relationship. Building it is the first and perhaps central task of the therapy, even for therapists who use a model in which the therapeutic relationship is not a focus.

Showing interest and communicating real empathy are examples of how beginning therapists can use themselves effectively in therapy and begin to build a relationship. Empathy—the ability to enter into a client's subjective world and to use one's own life experiences, thoughts, and feelings in relating to the client's pain—creates a powerful bond between the therapist and client and often builds an intimate relationship. Because of this profound connection, therapists must take the responsibility to conduct themselves appropriately with their clients. They need not "take on" the experience of their client to be empathic. The pain belongs to the client, not the therapist. The therapist shares the burden in relieving the difficulties, not in carrying them.

In our experience, there is also some truth to the idea of "fit" between client and therapist. Some therapists will be a good match with particular clients and some will not. A strong lack of fit might signal the therapist to offer a referral to someone else, or to suggest that the client shop for another therapist. In either case, the capacity of the therapist to empathize with the client is a relational quality basic to building the therapeutic alliance.

When one is working with a couple or family, empathy becomes more complicated. The therapist may relate strongly to one member and not to another. These emotional dynamics affect the connections within the clinical session and can be positive or negative contributors to treatment.

Allowing for a variety of empathic attachments within the clinical relationship taxes the therapist emotionally. Beginning family therapists often experience "combat fatigue" during their early work. Some interns think that separating family members and seeing them individually will help the family, but this strategy is just a way of trying to protect one's emotional energy. Learning how to create appropriate emotional boundaries with a client is essential for solid work. The ability to stay outside the system while maintaining some emotional attachment to its members is a delicate balancing act for the therapist. Supervision can provide feedback about this balancing, including a number of signs that indicate lack of it, such as going over the session time limit, responding to frequent client phone calls without setting clearer and more stringent guidelines for crisis calls, becoming preoccupied by the client so much that it interferes with other areas of life (insomnia, or thinking about a client all the time), or feeling like you're the only one who can help the client (the savior complex).

Good therapists provide a nonthreatening and trusting climate in which their clients are invited to be honest and to change. Therapists need to communicate a warm and accepting stance even in the midst of looking directly at difficult problems that are impacting clients. For example, a client may warily watch his therapist's reaction when he discloses that he believes his mother may have molested him when he was a child. Ready for blaming or shaming reactions, clients closely monitor how trustworthy and safe the therapist will be.

Trust is primary. Clients often have been accused of being "bad" or "wrong" for feeling, thinking, or acting in certain ways. A basic and open acceptance of each person must be in place in order to develop a therapeutic alliance. Clients need to experience the therapist as coming alongside of them and assisting them, not recoiling from them.

Clients also need to know that the therapist will be honest and appropriately self-disclosing when needed. For example, if the therapist is functioning outside of his or her comfort zone about a particular issue, sometimes it may be necessary to let the client know this. Beginning marriage and family therapists often feel this way when they start to provide therapy. Rather than "faking it," being clear about one's status as a trainee, about being supervised, and about working as a team with the client can engender more trust. Of course, trainees need to remember that they, too, have training and expertise from their education, previous clinical exposure, and their own life experience to bring to the therapeutic relationship.

As in assessment, curiosity contributes to developing a positive relationship with clients. Especially when working with persons with different life experiences than one's own—such as differences in age or culture, for example—taking a learning posture will often be helpful. It is difficult to stereotype when one takes this position, as a case example illustrates. A Laotian family came into therapy because their 12-year-old had "run away," that is, stayed overnight with a friend her parents didn't know, without telling them. One of the authors asked the parents how 12-year-olds could spend time with their friends in Laos when they were growing up, since the therapist didn't know their culture very well. They commented that 12-year-olds spend time with their friends only at school and spend time only with their families outside of school. Families would also get together with other families, and then their children would play together. The therapist asked these parents if they had discussed any "legitimate" way for their daughter to spend time with her peers other than at school or at their home. After looking at each other, they answered that they had not. The daughter then shyly commented that sneaking out was the only way she could be with her friends. The therapist and family then created some new ways for the 12-year-old to spend time with friends (besides school and family gatherings) that the parents and adolescent could accept. Listening and being curious about your clients' stories doesn't end after the first session. Probing to elicit information about them and their perspectives will promote a safe, healing context for understanding and change.

BASIC COUNSELING SKILLS

The following section highlights several core skills useful for family therapists, although not unique to our profession; they encompass skills used by many types of psychotherapies.

Structuring

In their groundbreaking book *The Family Crucible*, Napier and Whitaker (1978) state the importance of therapists winning the "battle for structure." In other words, therapists, not clients, need to establish and communicate (verbally and nonverbally) the ground rules for the process and content of therapy beginning with the first contact. For example, who is going to attend the first session? Napier and Whitaker believed it was essential for all family members to be present from the beginning of therapy and refused to start therapy until all were present. Such an expectation offers the family an orientation to systems thinking (Weber & Levine, 1995). Few family therapists follow this rigid stance (Berg & Rosenblum, 1977), and instead most make the decision about who will attend on a case-by-case basis (Nichols & Everett, 1986). However, therapists need to be clear with themselves and their clients about who the client is—individual, couple, or family (Weeks, Odell, & Methven, 2005).

Although we're uncomfortable with the "battle" metaphor, we strongly believe in the idea of therapists assuming a leadership role with their clients and guiding them through the assessment and treatment process. It is the therapist's job to provide a structure, including a time, a place, and setting for clients to safely talk about their concerns. Basic responsibilities include being on time for therapy sessions, maintaining a professional posture in the relationship (including dress and demeanor), following through on information you promise to offer in therapy (such as psychoeducational resources or referrals), remembering to ask about homework assignments, and taking responsibility for structuring the therapeutic time together (ending on time, reviewing treatment goals as needed, stopping an escalating argument), all of which strengthen the working relationship.

The therapist is also responsible for the format of therapy, including rules for the communication process, such as each person having a turn to talk and be heard. In very chaotic or volatile cases, the therapist may need to closely monitor the communication to assist the family in developing more effective communication skills. He or she may choose to initiate discussion of how material from the sessions will be used outside therapy. Again, the therapeutic environment needs to include an umbrella of safety; it may be useful to suggest to clients that certain topics are best discussed in therapy, at least until the family develops more effective communication skills.

Using (and Not Using) Self-Disclosure

One aspect of structuring is to ensure that the relationship with the client is one-sided: the content of the therapy is about the client, therapeutic goals are about the client, and self-disclosure is generally done by the client. Instead of seeking mutuality in the relationship, the therapist cares for the client and focuses on his or her problems. However, therapists may choose to make certain self-disclosures in a therapeutic context.

Therapists' disclosure of personal information will vary according to each one's personal style. Personal style in self-disclosure may be indicated by how intimately therapists decorate their office (for example, with photographs of spouse and children) and how directly they answer a client's questions about their own family life.

A therapist should consider some of the following guidelines in determining level of self-disclosure:

1. The therapeutic relationship, like any relationship, takes some time to develop. It is more appropriate to talk more personally about yourself after you've known someone for a longer time.

2. Most therapists self-disclose more freely with children and adolescents. These clients tend to equate self-disclosure with a measure of trust. They will ask more personal questions than adults and appear to be curious about the therapist.

3. Therapist credibility may be enhanced by self-disclosure of information about one's educational or professional credentials.

4. A therapist should keep in mind that self-disclosure may impact each client differently. Some clients will be more comfortable with a professional distance in which self-disclosure is kept to a minimum, while others will prefer to know something about the therapist before they feel comfortable opening up about themselves.

5. A therapist should disclose only personal information that has been thought about and processed, and avoid current issues that are creating personal turmoil.

The therapist must consider the impact of self-disclosure on the client. Providing information about oneself such as educational background or professional training can be very helpful in joining with a client and increasing confidence in the therapeutic process. Sometimes clients will ask personal questions, perhaps about marital status or whether you have children, and this can also be helpful in joining and in creating rapport. A therapist can offer personal reactions or feelings to a situation, such as being concerned about a client's well-being, as a leading statement to help generate a reaction from the client. A therapist may offer a story about his or her life or something that happened to someone else in order to stimulate the client's thinking or provide an alternative perspective on an issue. However, the therapist may also get caught up in his or her own reactions to a client and share feelings inappropriately, which might indicate that the therapist has lost direction in the therapeutic process.

It's helpful for the therapist to understand his or her own intentions in self-disclosing personal information and reactions, and attempt to anticipate the impact on the client. A couple coming to marital therapy may not benefit from knowing that their therapist is currently in the process of divorcing. In another case, it may be helpful for the therapist to normalize a couple's difficulty in coping with new parenthood by discussing personal experiences. Clearly, the degree to which a therapist's role encompasses sharing is driven by a combination of personal preference, theoretical orientation, and client considerations.

Although this discussion has been devoted to the therapist's responsibilities, remember that clients carry some responsibility as well—for their behavior and for making their own decisions. The therapist's role is to guide clients, not to make decisions for them. If a client decides to enter into a relationship that may be personally destructive, that decision needs to be respected by the therapist. He or she may offer alternatives or look at the client's motivation in entering into the relationship, but, ultimately, it is the client's choice. The client has to live with it. Finally, clients are responsible for bringing their concerns to therapy and maintaining some respect for the process. The therapy will likely be more productive if the client comes prepared to talk about issues of current concern.

Using Questions

From the first phone call, the therapist must use good questions in order to discover needed clinical information. Especially in the early and middle parts of the therapeutic relationship, questions keep the therapy focused on the client's perceptions and needs. In an effort to clarify the kinds of questions that can be used and the impact of specific types, Tomm (1988) reviews four categories of questions used in uncovering and understanding possibilities for treatment. All questions are seen as having a purpose, an intent.

Figure 6.1 denotes four types of questions: lineal, circular, strategic, and reflexive. *Lineal questions* are investigative, deductive, and content-loaded, involving a "just the facts, ma'am" perspective. Information gathered by these questions is thought to explain the problem. For example, questioning about why a child is truant and coming home late may be answered with "He doesn't like it; he hates the teachers; he hates the kids; he didn't like school last year, either; he needs an attitude adjustment." Often lineal questions point to something or someone who is "wrong" and needs to be fixed.

Circular questions are exploratory and stem from a posture of curiosity on the therapist's part. Instead of singling out who or what needs changing, information from these questions highlights interconnections within the family and to larger systems. Underlying the questions is the assumption that everything is connected to everything else.

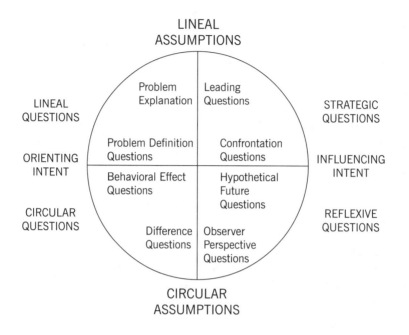

FIGURE 6.1. Question grid. From Tomm (1988, p. 12). Copyright 1988 by the Family Process Institute. Reprinted by permission of Blackwell Publishing Ltd.

A therapist might ask, "What, if anything, is different about the days when your son doesn't cut school?" or "Who in the family first finds out that your son has cut school? What happens after?" Circular questions help to expose patterns in the relationships.

O'Brian and Bruggen (1985) have classified circular questions into four different categories. One type of question has a family member comment on the relationship or interaction between two other family members. For example, the therapist may ask the mother, "How do your son and husband get along?" Or the therapist may ask a child, "What does your mother do when your father comes home and has been drinking?" Another type of circular question may have individuals rank-order family members' responses to an actual or hypothetical situation. A therapist might ask, "Who is most upset about the divorce? Who next?" Or he might ask more generally, "Who will be most relieved when this problem is resolved? Who will be next most relieved?" A third type examines differences that occur over time. Questions can relate to a specific event that happened in the past or is anticipated to happen in the future. For example, a mother might be asked how her child's behavior has changed since the divorce, or a father might be asked how his marriage will change once the children leave home. A fourth type of circular question is used to solicit information indirectly about an individual who is unwilling to answer questions or is not present. A wife may be asked by the therapist, "If your husband were here today, what would he say are the biggest problems in your marriage?"

A third category on the question grid presented in Figure 6.1 consists of *strategic questions,* or influencing questions, which are challenging in nature. They pose new possibilities, often in a particular direction. A therapist might ask, for example, "What would it take to have you and your ex-husband take a united parental stand with your child on this matter?" or "What might happen if you and your child's father ignored your child's behavior of leaving school early for a few weeks?" In both questions the therapist attempts to interrupt the current interactional sequence by having the parents align their behavioral reactions to their child. The question is purposive and often corrective. Changing the way the family currently responds to a problem is primary when asking strategic questions.

Reflexive questions facilitate change in the family without moving the family in any particular direction. Therapists, through their questions, attempt to mobilize new response possibilities from the family. The therapist assumes clients have and can access internal resources for change. Examples of reflexive questions are "What if your son had some strong feelings that he couldn't share with you, how could you let him know that you wanted to hear them?" or "If your son started attending school regularly again, how would your lives be different?" In both examples, a fairly neutral stance is taken by the therapist, in the belief that the client can find new responses that are "different and better" than previous responses. Rather than focusing on any precise behavior change, the door is opened to alternatives. Reflexive questions facilitate change without directing it.

In all these types of questions, nonverbal as well as verbal skills communicate the posture and perspective of the therapist. For example, a question like "What is your reaction?" can be asked in a demanding or a requesting way. Keeping nonverbal communication and verbal questions congruent allows more effective communication. In any case, the skill of questioning contributes to our ability to act as agents of change in the lives of the families we serve.

Normalizing

Normalizing requires some knowledge of what's common for many families to experience. It means that the therapist understands the symptoms presented by a client as part of common behavior connected with particular developmental phases in an individual's or a family's life. Framing a 14-year-old's moodiness as "a common part of adolescence" often helps relieve a family's concern. Normalizing a couple's distress over decreasing romantic interest while they have two preschool-age children can help them accept and understand rather than fear the changes in their relationship. Often a therapist notices an immediate calming in the client system when something has been normalized. Sometimes the family will respond by offering up stories that validate the normality of the symptoms (e.g., when Uncle John had the same problem).

Providing psychoeducational resources such as developmentally sensitive books or self-help groups and readings can be quite helpful for normalizing problems. We have included in this text discussions about normative reactions to life cycle and other developmental issues. Self-help groups also provide a strong normalizing experience for clients, especially those who are more socially isolated. For some, committing to a very short-term treatment contract (three to five sessions) helps to reassure the family that their concerns are interpreted as normal, and sets the appropriate clinical tone for the family. After brief therapy, one can reevaluate if the problem has been adequately addressed after labeling symptoms as normal. Many good developmental texts are available to clinicians to assist in normalizing.

Reframing

Sometimes change can occur through cognitive shifts rather than behavioral shifts. Reframing relies on the therapist's creative ability to reinterpret symptoms presented in therapy. Normalizing is one type of reframing since it attempts to decrease the anxiety about a particular problem by viewing it as normal.

Reframing allows clients to see their issues from another point of view, thus opening up the possibility for new responses. For example, a single mother comes into therapy because of the temper tantrums displayed by her 6-year-old daughter. The mother views this behavior as "willful disobedience and attempting to get her own way." Upon review of the circumstances often accompanying the tantrums, the therapist notes that the child gets very little undivided attention from her mother and then reframes the child's tantrum as a desire to "get more attention from Mom" and a "crying out since she feels lonely inside." Reframing the child's behavior in this way may change the ways the mother responds to her child. New ways the child might receive support from her mother can be considered.

Providing Support

As our society becomes more and more transient, providing a stable, consistent, and nurturing relationship in a client's life often resembles throwing a life jacket to a drowning person. The key way that therapists provide this nurturance is through attentive and active listening to the client's story. As the therapist begins to reflect back, understand, and grant permission to explore any and all feelings or thoughts, clients experience reassurance, a solid foundation from which to build new possibilities. "Just being there" makes a difference.

Yet support, however valuable, does not guarantee change. With the sweeping influence of healthcare reform and the need to justify each dollar spent on mental health care, supportive psychotherapy appears to be in question, regarded almost as a luxury. Support is more stabilizing in function than change inducing. Providing a reassuring place to be might not address the problem presented by the client. It must be remembered that clients usually don't seek therapy when everything is great, but rather when they are experiencing pain. This pain signals something significant and must be respected. Support can help to alleviate some of the pain but often won't remedy it. Change resulting from a supportive stance can be dramatic but often requires a long-term relationship, perhaps 1 or 2 years, before results are seen.

If you wish to explore some of the theoretical ideas behind a supportive posture in therapy, readings in the self psychology, attachment theory, and person-centered literature will be valuable. We recommend *Treating the Self* (Wolf, 1988) and *On Becoming a Person* (Rogers, 1972).

Confronting

To facilitate change, at some point during the therapy clinicians need to ask clients if they really want to change. This may or may not be done directly. Some therapies based on strategic models spend little time providing verbal support (although they do provide nonverbal support) and jump right into the domain of confrontation by using strategic or reflexive questions. For example, the first question from a solution-focused therapist might be "What would need to happen during our first session today to help with the problem you called about?" A change posture is expected and clients will be "fired" from therapy if they are unable to respond to change-oriented probing. Confrontation, although delivered with sensitive and concerned words, may begin immediately.

For some therapists and some clients, beginning therapy with a more confrontive posture won't be fitting. These therapists and clients must discover the appropriate time to move into more change-focused activities. Of course, this might be done sooner than one thinks. For example, as soon as a therapist develops an intelligent treatment plan, he or she necessarily moves into the confrontive domain since the treatment plan identifies specific areas to change. Likewise, as soon as the therapist wonders if involving other family members might help the situation, he or she is confronting the status quo. When a therapist tries to evaluate if therapy is helping, he or she moves into doing something different. Confrontation is essential to change.

Systemically oriented therapists know something about the difficulty we have in facilitating change. We know that clients tend to maintain homeostasis—the familiar way of handling a problem. Change takes energy and is often difficult to achieve. Directly or indirectly, the therapist must confront old ways of doing things and seek new possibilities in order for change to occur.

Pacing

The pace at which a therapy session moves involves how slowly or rapidly material is revealed by the client. The therapist's interventions can alter the pace by creating opportunities for further exploration of a particular issue, changing the focus to another topic, adding depth or breadth to the discussion, or exploring the emotions related to the issue. All of these interventions will impact what clients reveal and will lead them in a particular direction. Most interventions will be focused on either pacing or leading the client or family. In its simplest form, pacing involves "following the client." Mirroring a client's behavior enables the therapist to move at the client's pace. Techniques such as reflecting, active listening, and tracking also provide useful vehicles for pacing. Pacing a client is an essential aspect of the joining process and is critical in developing rapport and building a trustful, working relationship.

Leading is an attempt by the therapist to select a direction for exploration and lead the client there. Joining with the client must precede moving to a leading stance. If a young man is talking about his concerns about going to college, the therapist might first pace the client's concerns by listening to him. The therapist can then lead him by asking questions regarding his feelings about college and his thoughts about his ability to be successful. The introduction of the new focus expands the breadth and depth of the discussion and leads the client in a particular direction.

The therapist should monitor the pace of the session. If too much material is revealed too rapidly, there might not be sufficient time to follow up on critical events or issues, or the family's emotional response to a particular concern may be obscured. Slowing down the pace of the session often proves helpful in allowing clients to follow their own belief or feeling about an issue. If the pace is too slow, clients or therapists can become complacent and bored with the session. The therapist may need to intervene to move the session along by asking thought-provoking questions or focusing on present, here-and-now behavior. Most sessions will alternate between some pacing of the concerns and some leading to assist in developing alternative directions to be explored.

Several factors should be considered in determining the pace of therapy. If the family is highly motivated to change, then the pace of the therapy can be more rapid. High levels of resistance will likely mean that the pace will be slower. The length of treatment is also a factor. Brief therapy may limit the depth of exploration. The client's level of anxiety will also be a consideration in developing the pace. If anxiety is high the therapist may need to slow things down to assist in containing the client's fears. If the client's anxiety is extremely low there may be a lack of motivation to change, and the pace may need to be increased.

Specific techniques that hasten the pace of therapy include asking open-ended questions, leading in a particular direction, identifying the process in the session, and focusing on the here and now. Techniques that slow down the pace include tracking and obtaining clarification, mirroring behavior, active listening, and reflecting.

Dealing with Crises

Sometimes therapy begins with a crisis, a situation made up of unique circumstances that tend to be short term, overwhelming, and understandably stressful. Sudden and unexpected external events such as the death of a family member, an automobile accident, or a natural disaster are examples of events that could cause a client to be under severe stress or "in crisis." Crisis can occur around developmental or maturational issues such as the birth of a child, a child reaching adolescence, or the last child leaving home. Each individual or family will react to the situation differently and cope with it idiosyncratically. The crisis state is characterized by severe disruption in the client's or family's normal level of functioning. Common symptoms include physical and psychological agitation, poor appetite, loss of sleep, emotional distress, anxiety, and an inability to solve problems. Although the objective reality of a crisis such as a natural disaster may be the same to most people, responses to the event are highly subjective. A client's level of vulnerability will depend upon his or her subjective interpretation of the event, available resources, and previous history in coping with stress. When a crisis involves suicidal or homicidal ideation, child abuse, or elder or dependent adult abuse, we must not only attend to the needs of the client, but also act swiftly to carry out our ethical and legal responsibilities.

Even within a family each person will respond to a crisis differently, which can exacerbate family difficulties. For example, a family was about to go to court to settle a case involving an automobile accident in which their 17-year-old son was at fault. The event was causing a severe amount of stress for the parents, who had an exhaustive argument prior to the court appearance in which they both became very caustic and verbally abusive. The potential threat to their already unstable financial picture caused considerable fear and insecurity. The parents' response to the upcoming court hearing was to become agitated and conflictual, while the young man's response was to withdraw and deny the importance of the problem. Their reactions caused further difficulties between the family members, and thus a situational crisis ensued.

Families respond in their characteristic ways to a potential crisis. A crisis may escalate very quickly in a family in which anticipation of a worst-case scenario adds to the problem. In another family a crisis can be avoided through use of effective problem-solving skills. The family's ability to respond to a crisis will depend upon their ability to handle stress and conflict.

Crisis intervention tends to be short term and present focused. The therapist typically needs to assume an active and directive role in assisting clients when they are under severe stress. Rappaport (1970) has identified four goals for crisis intervention:

1. Relieving the client's immediate symptoms.
2. Restoring the client to his or her previous level of functioning.
3. Identifying the factors that led to the crisis state.
4. Identifying and applying remedial measures.

Crisis intervention techniques will vary, depending upon the client's state and the nature of the crisis. Affective interventions will focus on assisting the family in expressing their feelings about the situation, as often there is little opportunity to do so during the actual event. A debriefing period should allow clients to express their feelings and the therapist to provide support for what the family has been through. Normalizing their response to the situation may also be helpful. Cognitive interventions may focus on altering negative beliefs, guilt, or self-incriminating thoughts. For example, if a family is involved in an accident in which one member dies and another lives, assisting the surviving member in alleviating guilt may be an important initial intervention. By providing an opportunity to take action, behavioral tasks can help the client begin to regain a sense of control over his or her life. Beginning to rebuild shortly after a disaster can prove helpful in coping with psychological and material losses. Assisting the family in using community resources from agencies, churches, synagogues, or social programs may also be valuable.

Offering Psychoeducational Information

Another basic resource that can be developed by therapists is verbal and written information that can be provided to family members about common presenting problems. Develop a handout file for clients on common topics such as "Communication Skills," "Attention-Deficit/ Hyperactivity Disorder," "Depression," "Helping Your Adolescent," "Basics in Parenting," or "Alcoholism," or compile a book list of useful self-help books on various topics. The division between academic information and self-help references has become blurred in recent years, and many wonderful books and articles are available to help families with particular life issues.

INTERVENTIONS UNIQUE TO THE SYSTEMIC FAMILY THERAPIST

What do most family therapists do to create change? The empirical and clinical literature has attempted to answer this question, which has led to the development of many integrative models (e.g., Lebow, 2004), the exploration of common factors in family therapy (Miller, Duncan, & Hubble, 1997; Sprenkle & Blow, 2004), and the identification of core family therapy techniques (Seaburn, Landau-Stanton, & Horwitz, 1995). The relational and systemic models of family therapists provide a unique perspective on achieving change. Below, we identify and define 10 interventions that are commonly employed by family therapists.

Altering the Hierarchy

Hierarchy refers to the way leadership is organized in the family (Nichols & Schwartz, 2007). During assessment, a therapist might observe that the parents and children have equal power (flat hierarchy) or the children have more power than the parents (incongruous hierarchy). A common example is that of a parentified child: A child becomes part of the spousal subsystem and takes on an inordinate amount of responsibility, including caring for the emotional well-being of his or her parents (Nichols & Everett, 1986). When therapists alter the hierarchy, they are usually attempting to empower a parent or parents to take on a stronger leadership position in the family. It could also mean helping the parents form a less permeable boundary around their relationship and repositioning children, such as those who have been parentified, in the sibling subsystem.

Boundary Making

Boundary making allows the therapist to open or close boundaries between subsystems or between the family and other social systems, such as the school system. A therapist achieves the goal of boundary making, for example, when he or she intervenes to make sure each family member has uninterrupted time to speak or rearranges the chairs in the room to mark a boundary. For example, a therapist might ask a child sitting between his parents to move to another seat, allowing the therapist to more clearly define the spousal subsystem.

Enactment

Enactment is used for both assessment and treatment. For assessment purposes, a therapist uses enactment to observe family interactions by asking the family to reenact a specific problematic event or discuss a specific topic. As an intervention, enactment allows the therapist to directly alter family relationships by interrupting negative interaction and moving it in a more positive direction (Butler, Davis, & Seedall, 2008).

Exploring Exceptions to Presenting Problems

This intervention provides insight to the therapist and family about moments when the problem does not exist. The details of these moments may give information about what a family is doing competently to manage a problem, which can provide encouragement and hope.

Externalizing Problems

Externalization, a technique from narrative therapy, separates the problem from the person, thus giving the family an opportunity to join together with the therapist to address the influence of the problem.

For example, an initial step in externalization is giving the problem a name and then working on the relationship between the client and the problem.

Genogram Development

For assessment purposes, a genogram is a visual map to identify members of a family, including gender, generation, and age. As an intervention, a genogram becomes a focal point away from the presenting problem to help clients appreciate the larger context of their challenges, such as family themes and intergenerational relationship patterns.

Identifying and Interrupting Negative Interactional Patterns

Family therapists identify relationship patterns by observing families and carefully listening for interactional themes in detailed problem descriptions. To interrupt negative interactional patterns, therapists address the behavioral, cognitive, and emotional domains of family relationships. For example, emotionally focused therapists will identify and label primary emotions (e.g., hurt) underneath secondary reactive emotions (e.g., anger) to soften the interactions between family members and interrupt negative patterns.

Identifying Family Strengths

Presenting problems are frequently saturated with details about deficits. Identifying family strengths gives the therapist and family an opportunity to discover, or rediscover, positive qualities about individuals within the family and the family as a whole. Like problems, strengths have a history to be explored and understood.

Inviting Absent Family Members to Sessions

It's quite rare for an entire family to arrive for the first therapy appointment. More commonly, therapists initially make contact with part of a system, such as an individual, couple, or parent and child. Most systemic family therapists attempt to engage family members who do not participate in the first or second session, either by asking the client to invite other family members to a session or by the therapist contacting family members directly to seek their involvement. For example, if a mother and child present to therapy due to the child's unwillingness to attend school, a therapist might ask for the father's involvement at subsequent sessions.

Timeline Development

Like a genogram, a timeline helps clients place their concerns in context. A timeline records the significant normative events (e.g., transition to adolescence) and non-normative events (e.g., unexpected job loss) in a family's life. For example, a family might learn that a child's problem behavior began at a time of increased family stress during several concurrent transitions, including the arrival of a new sibling and a move to a new home and school.

BECOMING MORE SOPHISTICATED IN USING INTERVENTIONS

In addition to using basic counseling skills and intervening systemically, family therapists must consider issues of process and content, timing, and clients' anxiety levels when selecting specific interventions.

O'Hanlon (1982) has identified 13 classes of intervention that delineate different options for intervening in personal and interpersonal patterns of behavior, perception, and experience. These interventions are focused on altering patterns of behavior as they affect symptoms. For example, if the family presents constant arguing as the problem, the intervention is used to disrupt the pattern by altering how often arguments take place.

Interventions can focus on the process or content of a dialogue or interaction. The content of an interaction is what is actually said, while the process is how it is said (Satir, 1967). For example, a father and his 15-year-old son might be discussing the young man's desire to get his driver's license. This issue is the content, or *what* is being discussed. The process, or *how* it is being discussed, includes underlying feelings of concern, the tone of the discussion, and the communication pattern. Interventions that focus on content help to clarify issues, provide more information, and define problems. Interventions that focus on process aid in exploring or uncovering feelings and revealing themes or patterns of interaction. For example, if the therapist notices that family members are discussing a very emotionally charged issue with an absence of feeling, the therapist might intervene to identify this process. Solid therapeutic interventions involve both content and process.

A therapist considers several critical factors when choosing interventions. The timing of the intervention must be considered in evaluating its effectiveness. Timing affects how a particular strategy, a homework assignment, or a directive will be received by the family. Using a particular intervention too early in therapy, when there is insufficient trust in either the therapist or the process, can cause it to fail.

In addition to trust, it is helpful to consider motivation for change in determining appropriate timing. If a client is highly motivated, he or she likely will be more receptive to interventions that accentuate change. If the client is resistant to change, then interventions that pace the client, such as tracking and active listening, might be in order. In the initial therapy session, where the primary goal is assessment, a "no change" stance can be beneficial. The "no change" stance assumes that until the therapist has completed an adequate assessment, introducing change is premature. It really does not make good therapeutic sense to suggest change before fully comprehending the problem.

Assessing and managing anxiety in a session can prove helpful in evaluating the choice of an intervention. Some interventions, such as open-ended questions, can increase a client's anxiety simply because the client doesn't immediately know the answer. Questions that are more orienting in nature, such as basic information regarding family or work history, are likely to decrease anxiety. A moderate level of anxiety is to be expected in therapy and assist in moving toward change. It is helpful for the therapist to note the level of anxiety in the session and anticipate which interventions are likely to heighten or diminish it.

CONCLUSION

The basic treatment skills discussed in this chapter must be coordinated with the art of matching these skills to particular clients with particular problems, keeping in mind the kind of therapist you are. This is a lifelong and challenging component of being a family therapist. Good therapy is like good art—basics need to be mastered first: understanding yourself, your clients, and your context at multiple levels provides the setting in which a masterpiece is created. We close this chapter on treatment skills by offering, in Table 6.1, a list of self-assessment questions. Beginning therapists may find these helpful in gauging and guiding their early work.

TABLE 6.1. Self-Assessment Questions Regarding Treatment Skills

<u>To create a therapeutic relationship</u>

1. Do I show a concerned interest for my clients?
2. Have I structured a safe therapeutic environment in the room and set guidelines for working outside of the session?
3. Can I understand my clients' experience to some extent at both emotional and cognitive levels?
4. Do I continue to be curious about this case?
5. Do I need to be clear about my status as a trainee or intern, or my lack of expertise in a particular area?

<u>To assess and intervene</u>

1. Do I ask the appropriate questions to assess (e.g., lineal and circular questions) and intervene (e.g., strategic and reflexive questions)?
2. Can I normalize the clients' concerns in some way?
3. Will reframing the presenting problem help to change the way it is understood?
4. Do the clients perceive me as increasing their social support system?
5. Can I confront the family when necessary?
6. Am I aware of the pacing needs for these clients?
7. Have I considered referrals that would be useful?
8. Would psychoeducational material (e.g., reading, handouts, Internet website) be useful for these clients?
9. Do I have a treatment plan in place?

<u>To develop my family therapy skills</u>

1. Am I thinking and acting in a systemic manner?
2. Do my interventions match my systemic understanding of the problem and family?
3. Would it be useful to read an article or chapter on this treatment approach or problem? Do I need to attend a workshop to deepen my understanding?
4. Do I consult with a colleague or supervisor if I get confused?
5. Am I managing the legal and ethical concerns of this case well?

CHAPTER 7

Working with Families and Children

Lisa S sat wide-eyed and trembling on the edge of her chair, occasionally hiding with one hand a persistent tic in her left eye. It was her first visit to a therapist's office, and since 9-year-old Lisa was by nature a shy and nervous child, she left the talking to her mother and father. Mr. and Mrs. S leaned toward the therapist, and painfully revealed their daughter's daily panic attacks and their own frustration in trying to solve Lisa's "problem." By the end of the interview, the therapist had compiled a rich history and a number of hypotheses about Lisa's disorder. Although Lisa was clearly the IP, there was no question that family work would be part of treatment. Having carefully listened to and empathized with his new clients, the therapist began to talk teamwork . . .

Perhaps our deepest conviction in working with children is that, with remarkably few exceptions, primary caretakers are absolutely key to the assessment and effective treatment of childhood disorders. This "umbrella" assumption is a common value of family therapists, but is at times not put into practice by new therapists who feel anxious involving multiple family members. We hope you will consider the following:

1. Without caretakers as cotherapists, our interventions with children may become 50-minute exercises whose impact quickly dissipates in the 10,000 minutes that lie between sessions.
2. Whether we lean toward a view of childhood problems as somehow functional within the family or are inclined to see childhood disorders from a more individual perspective, our work

with children almost always involves addressing the hopes, fears, attitudes, and abilities of the grownups with whom our child clients live. Indeed, a collaborative set in which parents or primary caretakers share their own "assessments" and carry insights, information, and actions learned in therapy into the home is basic.

With this single principle to guide us, we present in this chapter a brief discussion of assessment issues with children, recent research findings regarding family interventions, and some pointers for working with children and their families at various life cycle and developmental stages. Finally, we complete the chapter with comments regarding special considerations for divorcing and remarried families, mediation and child custody evaluation, and the challenges of helping disadvantaged single-parent families.

ASSESSMENT OF CHILD AND ADOLESCENT DISORDERS

Art historians are likely familiar with that period of time in which European painters depicted children as miniature adults. Similarly, sociologists and anthropologists report on those eras in which children were surmised to think, feel, and behave as adults in undersized bodies. Today, of course, the differentiation between "child" and "adult" is as complex as it is well documented. In psychopathology, however, we continue the struggle to define, identify, and treat mental disorders that, previously described and treated among adults, behave quite differently in children.

In our work in an inpatient psychiatric facility for children, we are reminded daily of how childhood itself complicates differential diagnoses (Costello, Mustillo, Erkanli, Keeler, & Angold, 2003; Hofstra, Van der Ende, & Verhulst, 2000). The common behavioral symptoms seen in troubled children cut across neat diagnostic categories and, in so doing, engage all our skills of assessment and appropriate treatment planning: "Are this child's mood swings a sign of ADHD? Bipolar disorder? Should a DSM-IV-TR diagnosis even be made? Or are these symptoms an offshoot of marital conflict and 'poor parenting'?" In any case, diagnoses are made with caution, and assessment is ongoing and comprehensive, involving biological evaluations (e.g., electroencephalograms [EEGs] and magnetic resonance imaging [MRI] to detect brain abnormalities), as well as social (detailed information gathering regarding family, school, and peer relationships) and psychological ones (use of paper-and-pencil instruments and projective tests).

While a biopsychosocial approach enriches our assessment of childhood *and* adult disorders, we cannot overestimate the importance of assessing family issues, particularly when the IP is a youngster. Estrada and Pinsof (1995) point out the growing influence of a systems view in child assessment by noting the following common premises: (1) the view of child and family disorders as constellations of interrelated systems and subsystems; (2) the need to consider the entire family situation when assessing the impact of any single variable; (3) the idea that similar behavior may be the result of different sets of initiating factors; (4) a recognition that intervention is likely to lead to multiple outcomes, including readjustment of relationships within the family system; and (5) the notion that family systems and subsystems possess dynamic properties and are constantly changing over time (p. 405).

In addition, a growing body of literature suggests that the development of child and adolescent problems does not occur in a vacuum but is strongly influenced by certain marital and family characteristics (Achenbach, 2008; Essex et al., 2006). For example, factors such as marital discord, parental psychopathology, social-cognitive deficits in family members, socioeconomic disadvantage, disrupted parent–child relations, lack of social support, and social isolation are all variables that strongly influence the course of a child's individual disorder. This literature gives a strong argument for a systemic assessment.

Having considered these important family variables, the therapist working with Lisa S and her parents would have discovered some enlightening facts and expanded his hypotheses for later treatment. We learn, for example, that Lisa's father has a history of panic attack and agoraphobia; that both parents are inadvertently maintaining Lisa's symptoms by avoiding using the words "death" and "dying," which often precipitate attacks; that Mr. S has unresolved grief issues from a death in his family; and that Mr. and Mrs. S disagree strongly about how to parent their daughter but avoid discussions or arguments about these differences. We also find that about the time Lisa's attacks began, her father had lost his job due to his agoraphobia and a role change had occurred in which Dad now stayed home to care for Lisa and Mom left the house to work.

Certainly, individual assessment and diagnosis of children is important. In Lisa's case, we can use DSM-IV-TR and find that our client meets the criteria for panic attacks. Based purely on individual symptoms reported by Lisa and her parents, we can then design a treatment program based on known effective interventions for anxiety disorders. However, by taking a systemic as well as an individual approach in our evaluation, we can supplement Lisa's treatment by addressing the family issues that clearly impact her symptoms. Thus, our assessment has expanded and enriched the treatment.

While family therapists are primarily concerned with systemic assessment and intervention, it will be increasingly important for all clinicians to have an up-to-date and working knowledge of individual diagnoses for children and adolescents. For example, a familiarity with such common childhood diagnoses as depression, behavioral disorders or ADHD, pervasive developmental disorders (autism), and conduct disorders is expected. Other problems that are frequently diagnosed in children and adolescents include fear and anxiety disorders (especially phobias) and substance abuse. Many children have problems that are comorbid. For example, a young child may be diagnosed with ADHD and later be diagnosed with a conduct disorder and substance abuse problem.

It is beyond the scope of this section to describe in detail the diagnostic criteria for each child and adolescent disorder. A brief summary is presented in Table 7.1.

Family therapists are well advised to become familiar with such instruments as the Child Behavior Checklist (see Conners, 1997), in which multiple sources provide information about a child's behavior, and the Conners' Rating Scales, a neuropsychosocial instrument for assessing hyperactive children (Conners, 1997). In addition, since child and adolescent assessment often focuses on development, many pencil-and-paper instruments and projective tests are used to assess intelligence and development, including the Wechsler Intelligence Scale for Children, 3rd edition (WISC-III; Wechsler, 1991), the draw-a-person test, and the house–tree–person tests (Buck & Jolles, 1966). Many of these tests are used in the educational batteries of school districts. While most family therapists will not be administering these instruments as part of their therapy, it is important that they know what psychological evaluation instruments are available and make appropriate referrals for further evaluation, especially when they suspect a child has a developmental disorder or other learning problem.

FAMILY INTERVENTIONS
WHEN CHILDREN ARE THE CLIENTS

Beginning therapists often struggle with how to do family therapy when the client is 7 years old and isn't inclined to disclose concerns or talk about feelings. While various forms of play therapy and other projective approaches help a child express or work through problems,

TABLE 7.1. Common Childhood Disorders

Category of disorder	Essential features
Attention-deficit/ hyperactivity disorder	1. Inattention: inability to finish activities that require concentration at school, home, or play; doesn't seem to listen; easily distracted. 2. Hyperactivity: excessive activity; fidgets excessively; can't sit still. 3. Impulsivity: impatience; difficulty waiting for one's turn; interrupts or intrudes excessively. 4. Behavioral manifestations occur in more than one setting, were present before age 7, and impair developmentally appropriate functioning.
Conduct disorder	1. Violation of basic rights of others, norms, or rules. 2. Behaviors includes some or all of the following: aggression toward people and animals; destruction of property; deceitfulness or theft; and serious violation of rules (truancy, running away).
Autism spectrum disorders	1. Impaired social interaction: eye contact is lacking; doesn't seek interaction. 2. Impaired communication: delay in, or lack of, speech; stereotyped use of language; idiosyncratic use of language. 3. Restricted, repetitive behaviors: abnormally intense preoccupation with object or activity; inflexible adherence to rituals or routine; repetitive motor movements.
Attachment disorders (separation anxiety and reactive attachment disorders)	1. In separation anxiety: excessive anxiety about being away from home or from person to whom child is attached; distress or worry about losing other; fear and/or reluctance about sleeping alone, going to school; nightmares. 2. In reactive attachment disorder: failure to thrive; pathogenic care (neglect); excessive inhibition, hypervigilance, or ambivalence in social interactions.
Learning disorders	1. Academic functioning lower than expected given an individual's age, intelligence, and education. 2. Interference with academic achievement or activities of daily living that require reading, mathematical, or writing skills. 3. Demoralization, low self-esteem, and deficits in socials skills may be present. 4. There may be underlying abnormalities in cognitive processing (e.g., deficits in visual perception, linguistic processes, attention, or memory). 5. Ten to 25% of individuals with conduct disorder, oppositional defiant disorder, ADHD, major depressive disorder, or dysthymic disorder also have learning disorders.

(cont.)

TABLE 7.1. *(cont.)*

Category of disorder	Essential features
Depression	1. Depressed or irritable mood: feelings of sadness, hopelessness, worthlessness, guilt. 2. Loss of interest in activities once enjoyed. 3. Loss of energy: fatigue, inability to concentrate. 4. Change in appetite: failure to make expected weight gains. 5. Change in sleep: insomnia or hypersomnia. 6. Recurrent thoughts of death: suicidal ideation.

we return to our guiding principle—effective therapy, especially with children, will rely on helping parents or caretakers become engaged in the process, clarify their own roles in the family, and become cotherapists who conduct their own interventions at home.

At times, parents are reluctant to participate in therapy and even more reluctant to examine their own roles in the family's problems. We've observed beginning therapists relinquish their understanding of the family's impact on the child, especially when the parents, physicians, and other clinical professionals adhere to an individual perspective on psychopathology. While we would never want to return to the days when parents were blamed for their children's schizophrenia or other problems, we are equally uncomfortable with parents who drop their children off for therapy and return an hour later. Regardless of how or if parents influenced the development of a child's problem, we are confident that parents can be part of a successful resolution. Thus, we encourage you to assess the roadblocks to parental involvement.

Often, parents do not understand their child's problem or how they might help. Thus, psychoeducation can be an important part of your work. In the era of the Internet and self-help, parents have often begun the process of self-education before they ever start therapy. If not, you can provide parents with educational resources. In addition, parents sometimes do not know how to advocate for their child or obtain the resources their child needs. Again, your role might be to help the parent help the child, for instance, by helping the parent work more effectively with the child's school. Finally, parents may be dropping a child or teen off for therapy because their own lives are overwhelming—emotionally, financially, or structurally. Try not to fall into the trap of feeling critical of the parents and internally aligning yourself with the child, thus subtly believing that you are the child's secret protector. Instead, search for an empathic understanding of the parent's life. What brought the mother to this place? In what ways does it make perfect sense that this dad does not want to be involved in his child's struggles at school? If you can genuinely develop empathy and understanding of the parents' struggles, you can begin to help them help their child.

Treatment of Child-Focused Problems

Much of the child treatment literature draws on the parent management training (PMT) model developed by Gerald Patterson at the Oregon Social Learning Center. This model was originally developed for work with antisocial youth but has now been applied to a range of childhood disorders. The underlying assumption of the model is that behavior problems are inadvertently developed and maintained by maladaptive parent–child interactions. Therapists teach parents to use specific skills when interacting with their children in order to promote prosocial behavior and to decrease deviant behavior (Estrada & Pinsof, 1995).

Among the common characteristics shared by all PMT treatments are the following: (1) The treatment is conducted by parents who directly implement procedures in the home; (2) parents learn to identify, define, and observe problem behavior; (3) the treatment sessions cover social learning principles including positive reinforcement, punishment, negotiation, and contingency contracting; (4) these strategies are taught through a prescribed set of therapy activities including modeling and role playing; and (5) the program's goal is development of specific parenting skills.

Estrada and Pinsof (1995) report that PMT is probably the most widely used family intervention in the treatment of childhood disorders. Their review of 20 years' worth of empirical research demonstrates these and other findings in the study of common disorders of children:

1. *Conduct disorders* (including oppositional defiant disorder): Family therapy, especially PMT, is an effective treatment for families of children with conduct disorders. Maintenance of these improvements is still an issue; continuation of the gains made appears to be moderated by other factors, such as marital distress, social isolation, or other variables. Kazdin (1997) states that PMT is one of the most encouraging treatments for children with conduct disorder.

2. *ADHD*: Family interventions, particularly PMT, improve child management skills. Parents report increased confidence, reduced stress, and improved family relationships. Research demonstrates a reduction in children's noncompliance and aggression rather than in core symptoms such as inattention, impulsivity, and overactivity. Research definitely supports the use of medication to treat ADHD.

Longer-term, combined behavioral–medication treatments have the most lasting effects.

3. *Fears and anxiety disorders*: Anxiety problems are the most common psychological problems reported by children, and many adults with anxiety disorders report their problems started in childhood. These disorders include school phobias and other phobias such as fear of the dark, of medical visits, and of separation from parents. Research yields tentative support for the efficacy of approaches that involve parents in the treatment of their children's fear and anxiety.

4. *Autism*: Autism is the only developmental disorder with a clear body of family-based research supporting its efficacy. Autism research focuses on training a child's parents to serve as teachers and therapists, and it suggests that families with autistic children can achieve lasting gains from family-based interventions. Families that fare the best have the least cognitively impaired children (mental retardation is common in children with autism). They also have parents who can participate in a demanding treatment program, as well as support from schools that encourage parent training efforts at home.

More recent reviews of the child treatment literature provide evidence for the efficacy of family-oriented cognitive-behavioral therapy, family oriented group cognitive behavioral therapy, and parenting training for the treatment of behavioral and emotional disorders in children (Northey, Wells, Silverman, & Bailey, 2003). The most important lesson to learn from this summary of literature is that the inclusion of parents leads to better outcomes for children and parents for some disorders, particularly anxiety and ADHD.

Treatment of Adolescent-Focused Problems

While treatment models for problems in childhood tend to be based on parent education, treatment models for problems during adolescence tend to be family therapy models focusing on family patterns that accompany behavioral problems (Sexton, Sydnor, Rowland, & Alexander, 2005). Functional family therapy (Alexander & Sexton, 2002), multisystemic therapy (Henggeler, Pickrel, & Brodino, 1999), brief structural strategic family therapy (Szapocznik et al., 1988; Szapocznik & Williams, 2000), and multidimensional family therapy (Liddle, 1992, 1999) are now at the forefront of treatment for common problems experienced by adolescents and their families. One of the factors that contributes to their appeal is the research evidence that supports their effectiveness. An adequate description of each model is beyond the scope of this book, but we hope you'll find ways to learn more about these models. Many community mental health centers are now adopting these treatment approaches and provide training for their clinicians.

Emerging Resources for Treating Children and Adolescents

While parents' support and family-based treatments can serve as the foundation for child and adolescent interventions, other new resources also offer hope. New knowledge from neuroscience points to the critical importance of attachment for brain development (Siegel, 1999). In addition, brain research has led to a new understanding of many disorders. For example, some research suggests that at least some types of ADHD may be simply a case of delayed brain development (Duncan et al., 2007; Shaw et al., 2007). Other research on ADHD examined family-based interventions since ADHD frequently occurs in multiple family members. For example, researchers have noted that conflict and hostility in families make ADHD symptoms worse. To alleviate stress and conflict in families with ADHD, families are being taught meditation and mindfulness skills (Baruchin, 2008).

As research in neuroscience continues, family therapists can be aware of resources and referrals for their clients. For example, children and teens with learning challenges might benefit from neuropsychological evaluations. Usually these evaluations assess intelligence, academic achievement, visual-motor skills, and emotional health. Skills such as the ability to pay attention, the ability to remember information, and the ability to decide and execute one's plan are all important domains of a neuropsychological evaluation. If parents or schools have concerns about a child's functioning in any of these areas, a neuropsychological evaluation can offer critical information to guide the treatment.

Psychotropic medications are growing in popularity as a treatment for children and adolescents. While medications sometimes offer relief to families that have tried other options, concerns still exist about using medications to treat child and adolescent problems. Questions about the influence of the medications on child development, especially brain development, remain. In fact, several mental health organizations have issued position papers suggesting that nondrug treatments be considered first. These treatments should include techniques that focus on the adults in a child's life, including parents and teachers (Carey, 2006).

Genetics and heritability are other areas of study that are influencing our understanding of children's and teens' problems. For example, mental health professionals know that disorders like autism and ADHD have high heritability, 76% for ADHD and 90% for autism. In addition, genetic researchers are interested in gene–environment interaction.

What type of environment influences gene expression? Stated more simply, what type of environment "turns on" the gene, and when does the environmental influence start? For example, researchers have suggested that maternal smoking correlates with more serious mental health symptoms. Thus, the impact of the environment starts in the womb.

What can family therapists take from this exciting new research? While a child's genetics won't change, therapists can influence the child's environment. Armed with new knowledge about the importance of a healthy family environment, family therapists can feel confident when they help families reduce stress, reduce conflict, and increase close bonds.

THE FAMILY LIFE CYCLE REVISITED

As family therapists, we're keenly aware that children and families, and the problems they cope with, need to be viewed within a variety of contexts. As mentioned briefly in Chapter 5, one significant context that needs to be understood when assessing and treating problems in childhood and adolescence is the family's stage of development and how it interfaces with the problems that exist in a family. Building on early studies of the family (Duvall, 1955) and applying this information to the needs of the family therapist, Carter and McGoldrick (1989) categorized the family life cycle into six stages with a key emotional process and several developmental tasks at each stage (see Table 7.2).

The systemic backdrop to these ideas stems from the assumption that the family must go through a second-order change at each developmental stage for its members to proceed in a healthy way. Second-order change necessitates a redefining of the family system in behavioral, cognitive, emotional, and relational domains. Carter and McGoldrick's version of the family life cycle gives special attention to the transitions between stages.

Families often present to a therapist when they are in the midst of a developmental transition. The family therapist hypothesizes that the presenting problem may have a lot to do with the family being stuck in its progress toward achieving a particular developmental stage. For example, a 14-year-old daughter of very controlling parents may start "acting out" by breaking curfew and hanging out at school with people the parents deem unacceptable. This behavior signals a difficulty in the family system's transition to the "family with adolescents" stage, where there is a need to increase the permeability of the family boundaries to include the teenager's growing independence.

TABLE 7.2. The Stages of the Family Life Cycle

Family life cycle stage	Emotional process of transition: Key principles	Second-order changes in family status required to proceed developmentally
1. Leaving home: single, young adults	Accepting emotional and financial responsibility for self	a. Differentiation of self in relation to family of origin b. Development of intimate peer relationships c. Establishment of self; work and financial independence
2. The joining of families through marriage: the new couple	Commitment to new system	a. Formulation of marital system b. Realignment of relationships with extended families and friends to include spouse
3. Families with young children	Accepting new members into the system	a. Adjusting marital system to make space for child(ren) b. Joining in childrearing, financial, and household tasks c. Realignment of relationships with extended family to include parenting and grandparenting roles
4. Families with adolescents	Increasing flexibility of family boundaries to include children's independence and grandparents' frailties	a. Shifting of parent–child relationships to permit adolescent to move in and out of system b. Refocus on midlife marital and career issues c. Beginning shift toward joint caring for older generation
5. Launching children and moving on	Accepting a multitude of exits from and entries into the family system	a. Renegotiation of marital system as a dyad b. Development of adult-to-adult relationships between grown children and their parents c. Realignment of relationships to include in-laws and grandchildren d. Dealing with disabilities and death of parents (grandparents)
6. Families in later life	Accepting the shifting of generational roles	a. Maintaining own and/or couple functioning and interests in face of psychological decline; exploration of new familial and social role options b. Support for a more central role of middle generation c. Making room in the system for the wisdom and experience of the elderly, supporting the older generation without overfunctioning for them d. Dealing with loss of spouse, siblings, and other peers and preparation for own death. Life review and integration.

Note. From Carter and McGoldrick (1989). Copyright 1989 by Allyn & Bacon. Reprinted by permission of Pearson Education, Inc.

The first task at each transitional stage is for the therapist to normalize what is going on in the family, framing many of the presenting problems as common and understandable. A therapist can use the life cycle information to connect more fully with the family, as it helps him or her to understand their dilemmas more completely. In normalizing, a therapist must be careful not to trivialize the pain, fears, and emotional power of these developmental shifts. When done well, normalizing can be offered as a first "gift" to the family from the therapist, toning down the emotional turmoil within the family. The therapist's expertise in understanding what the family is about helps establish a solid working alliance. Thus, life cycle information boosts the therapist's authority, which is especially helpful if he or she is significantly younger than the other adults in the therapy room.

Knowing the key emotional issues at each developmental stage provides guidance to the therapist. What must the family members manage effectively in each stage? Therapists can connect to family members' deeper emotional issues by using information about the family life cycle. For example, the key emotional transition for two individuals to make in forming a committed relationship or marriage is "commitment to a new system." Without a new system that cultivates a place for each partner to be included and respected, a kind of competition takes place wherein each person attempts to win the battle for dominion over a particular area of life, be it housecleaning, finances, or friendships. A therapist, aware of the necessary emotional transition, can direct the couple to find ways in which each person can be comfortable with a decision. The therapist facilitates the couple's transition from a "me" to a "we." Of course, there is no "right" way to transition from one stage to the next. Each family will be guided by its own family histories and the belief systems of its race, culture, and ethnicity.

Next, we explore some of the key themes in four stages of family development: (1) families with young children; (2) families with school-age children; (3) families with adolescents; and (4) launching children and later life. Applying this material in your therapy sessions means that you ask yourself a few key questions each time you assess a new family. Those questions include:

- What are normal developmental tasks for this family given their family life cycle stage?
- How might the family's presenting problems influence their abilities to successfully navigate the developmental tasks?
- How might the developmental tasks be influencing the family's presenting problems?

You might also want to consider the overlap between individual development, family development, and the presenting problems. Thus, you might ask yourself the following questions:

- What are normal developmental tasks for the *individuals* in this family?
- How might the individual needs and the family's developmental needs be influencing the family's presenting problems?

For example, a therapist saw a family consisting of a 19-year-old, a husband, and a wife. During high school, the 19-year-old had been diagnosed with an aggressive form of cancer. For several years, she endured painful, exhausting treatments and at times the family wondered whether she would survive. She had to quit school and the basketball team. Her mother became her primary support and they traveled to a city several hours away for treatments. The father worked harder to help cover the skyrocketing costs of the treatments.

When the mother and daughter came for therapy because they were having conflict over the daughter's wish to start college in a city two hours away, the daughter had been in remission for over a year. While the treatment had been successful, the illness had wreaked havoc on the family. The couple had ignored their marriage for several years while they focused on helping their daughter. Now, three years later, they found they had little in common. In contrast, the mother's life had evolved around her daughter's health needs and she had gradually given up her individual life and her relationship with her husband. As the daughter's health improved, she began to seek more autonomy, while her mother remained resistant to letting go—partially because she feared that if she wasn't watching carefully, the cancer might reappear and partially because she wasn't sure what to do with her own life now that her daughter no longer needed her constantly.

At the launching stage of the family life cycle, this family's normative transition had gone awry because of the demands of the cancer and its painful treatments. Thus, considering the family life cycle and the tasks of both individual development and family development helped the therapist create a nonpathologizing plan to help the family get back on track.

Families with Young Children

Frank and Laura were on the verge of divorce when they agreed, as a last resort, to give therapy a try. With their 19-month-old daughter in tow, it soon became apparent to the therapist that the couple's smooth sailing days had ended when they struck the rocky shores of new parenthood. Since the birth of their baby and Laura's 6-week maternity leave, the couple had continued their prebaby work schedule. The baby was put into quality home childcare, but Mom and Dad felt guilty about this and spent all of their evening hours and weekend time devoted to their little girl. Before long, chronic crankiness (of the parents, not the baby!) deteriorated into outright fighting. Frank and Laura had a hard time remembering why they married in the first place. Clearly, without a renegotiation of their adult "couple space," divorce looked imminent.

This couple's story is a reminder that marital issues are paramount in this stage of the family life cycle. New parents must take time and energy to develop an emotional attachment to the baby, as well as meet his or her physical needs. A family's response to the new baby can range from a "hardly noticing" to a "drop everything" stance. In the former, or closed boundary, stance, the parent or couple won't be able to meet the needs of a very dependent child since a baby requires significant family resources. Neglect of one form or another can result. On the "drop everything" end of the spectrum, a family opens its arms wide to the child at the expense of all other relationships, including the couple's own. Though well suited for the very early aspects of this stage, a child-centered family often struggles with the growing independence needs of its members at later stages of the family life cycle. Problems of marital distress or individual functioning (depression) could result.

Fights over childrearing, household tasks, and financial responsibilities are common at this stage. Particularly when couples haven't formed a new system in the previous stage of the family life cycle (the joining of families), the practical urgency and plentitude of stressors and decisions here can seem overwhelming. Gender issues often come to the forefront at this stage, too. Sue and Joe, who lived together for 5 years, had been separated for 2 weeks when they sought therapy. Their 4-year-old son and 2-year-old daughter were the motivation behind this move, yet as we explored what brought them in, the couple's children seemed to make up the major battleground. Both Sue and Joe needed to work in order to make their rent payments, but Sue resented this, saying that Joe didn't make as much money as he could in his sales work. Sue, whose mother stayed home until Sue was in sixth grade, longed to be able to do the same. Joe, raised by his mom in a single-parent household, believed Sue needed to work in order to provide their children with the house and yard he never had. Clashes about role expectations, especially gender role expectations, come to a powerful crescendo at this stage.

An understanding of these practical, emotional, and interpersonal issues that appear in families with very young children can guide therapeutic interventions and help new parents make a successful transition from one life cycle stage to the next.

While this early phase of family life brings more parents than children to therapy, therapists will occasionally meet with families whose IP is an infant or toddler. Three-year-old Jason came to therapy for repeated aggressive behavior against his 1-year-old sibling, for destroying toys and household belongings, and trying to climb out of a moving car. His single mother presented Jason to the therapist with a simple plea: "I don't know why he does it! But you've got to make it stop!" Clearly, how the therapist explores Jason's problems and ultimately how he or she treats them are limited by Jason's age.

Family therapists who work with very young children can base their initial assessment and treatment on the child's developmental stage. The literature on children's emotional, cognitive, and social development from infancy to adulthood is voluminous, and we would do a disservice to its scholars to encapsulate developmental theory here. While we encourage beginning therapists to learn about or refresh themselves on the needs and expectations of each stage of childhood and adolescence, our focus is on brief reminders about developmental issues and practical steps to take when a young child toddles into your office.

Armed with the knowledge that infants and toddlers require secure attachments in order to build a trustful orientation toward life, we can assess very young children in terms of their early attachments and the sense of autonomy they show, among other variables. Our knowledge about cognitive development also shapes our expectations: for example, realizing that "time out" can be understood by a toddler, while "telling the truth" is much less clear to someone who is 3 years old. In Jason's case, for example, we learned that frequent separations from his mother and maltreatment by intermittent caretakers marked this youngster's first years of life. Further, his mother's ignorance of the cognitive capabilities of her toddler likely made the situation at home more difficult. Lengthy "explanations" of why siblings should not be hit or thrown had little impact on Jason's aggressive behavior. Immediately, we have clues to the route family therapy can take—reestablishing a secure attachment between Jason and his mother, and helping this single parent learn appropriate methods of dealing with her child's behavior.

Beginning therapists can also benefit from a number of practical guidelines for working with very young children. These involve space, safety, shared responsibility, and expectations.

Space

Most therapy offices don't fit the needs of both adults and children. Traditional play therapy rooms may be too cramped or full of potential hazards (paint, clay) for an adult to relax. In contrast, adult-oriented rooms with immobile furnishings may paralyze and increase anxiety in children. Ideally, therapy rooms should accommodate full family interactions as well as provide separate spaces for play and for separating out family subsystems, if needed. A larger room, sparsely furnished with movable chairs and pillows, could accommodate all. It's also helpful to have play areas with toys that encourage interaction between children and adults (hand puppets, crayons and paper, simple games). All of these assist therapy.

Safety

Safety needs to be established during the therapy session, and everybody can help make this possible. Therapists need to check the therapy room and remove or "childproof" potentially dangerous items before the session starts. Parents often believe the therapist will take responsibility for setting limits and discipline during the session. It's helpful to assign the major responsibilities to the parents instead, using rules they have at home. This offers a way to strengthen the parental position in the family hierarchy and gives the therapist an opportunity to see how the family functions.

Shared Responsibility

Although setting a collaborative tone with most families is helpful, allowing for a flexible sharing of the work with young children is essential. Therapists need to be able to sit on the floor and play with the children when this activity is useful. Parents can take their child for a walk as a break when necessary. Often cotherapy teams can assist greatly in managing the subsystems of a particular family. One therapist can take a child into another room, while the other therapist works with the parent. Also, selecting session times that don't interfere with naps and mealtimes is helpful. Asking parents to bring a favorite toy might be useful, too. Finally, creatively dividing up the family system for different sessions over time—one oriented for a parent–child focus, one for parents only—can assist in better management of therapeutic goals.

Expectations

For children in particular, nothing is sacred about weekly, 50-minute therapy sessions. Shorter or longer sessions or meetings divided into smaller segments can help the therapist's work with a family. Toddlers, in particular, will rarely be able to sit for more than a few minutes of talk, necessitating the need for play therapy involving games, artwork, or storytelling. Action in the therapy session and participation between family members are also helpful for older children and adults. In addition, family therapy often makes sense as "brief therapy." After a longer intake/assessment session, for example, a therapist might offer several interventions to be tried out over several weeks and request that the family report the results at a later session. Home visits, too, can often result in very helpful information on ways of adapting the environment to alleviate problems with a young child. In short, flexibility and teamwork are crucial to working with families with very young children.

Families with School-Age Children

Family life cycle concerns at this stage are similar to the previous ones in that they reflect a need to adapt to change. What often differs at this stage is the expansion of the family's contact with larger social systems. If children have been in half-day preschool, the transition now is to full-day school. If children have been in full-day childcare, they now have full-day school and participation in sports activities after school and on weekends. Further, evaluation of the child now involves comparisons with peers, and the ability or inability of a child to "fit in" becomes more prominent. The school system connects intimately with the life of the family. Problems or successes at school can impact the family system.

During this and the previous stage, relationship issues with extended family are also renegotiated. What will be the role of the grandparents, aunts, uncles, and cousins? Previous issues within the family that haven't been resolved are revived during this time. For example, when molestation or other kinds of abuse have occurred in the family, fears and boundary concerns come to the fore. For parents, the issue in therapy may relate to contacts their children will have with relatives. Glenda presented to her therapist the dilemma of what to do when her mother invited her 8-year-old daughter to spend the night for a weekend. Glenda had been molested by her stepfather, who was still married to her mother. She had an ongoing relationship with her family, but always watched her daughter when Grandfather was around. Glenda had worked on her past in group therapy but hadn't brought up her concerns to her family directly. Family therapists will frequently be called upon to help clients navigate transgenerational difficulties at this stage.

For the children in this stage, the focus is around starting school, moving out into the world, and building self-esteem by managing their environment more intentionally. Feelings of being a failure or success permeate activities such as tying shoelaces and learning to read. Development of initiative versus guilt and industry versus inferiority provide the basis of many daily concerns for the child. Peer relationships become more and more central, and comparisons to others—"Tommy's the best kickball player at school" or "June can read two books a day"—seem to pervade many social interactions. The task for parents, teachers, and therapist is to find places where a child can experience competency and some level of proficiency. If this is not the case at school, parents can look to sports, art, music, and relationships outside school for experiences that will help a child develop a healthy self-concept.

It's not surprising to find therapy clinics brimming with 5-, 6-, and 7-year-old children whose first months at school have been met with frustration or failure. This is the time when problems with attention, hyperactivity, anxiety, oppositionalism, and learning become evident to those outside the family. Frequently, young children make their way into therapy on the recommendations of schoolteachers and counselors. In some cases, the mere suggestion by school authorities is all the impetus distraught parents need to finally seek help.

This is an important point for beginning therapists to remember. By the time parents bring their youngsters to therapy, they are well acquainted with their child's behavioral problems and have likely tried "every trick in the book" to solve them. It's not unusual for us to see parents who report being fed up, exhausted, angry, lost, guilty, and in myriad other states when they arrive in our offices. Frequently, these beleaguered parents want you—the therapist—to fix the problem. Returning to our guiding principle, however, we're reminded that without the parent as cotherapist, our chances of success are minimal. Our first task, then, is to support and join with the parents, to empathize with their struggle, and to enlist their expertise as we present the real need for a team approach. Whether the treatment plan focuses on PMT (as is typical with problems involving very young children) or is combined with re-creating parent–child bonds and nurturing the warm relationships that often get lost in stressful circumstances, our ability to engage and work with parents is at the heart of therapy with these children.

At the same time, our sense is that therapy will progress further, and parents will commit more to the process, if we can creatively engage children at these ages—they are therapeutic allies, information resources, and affective conduits for the family. Probably the easiest way to involve children at this age is through drawing and role playing. Therapists who aren't able to create a child-centered therapy room can often hide a large art pad and markers for artistic purposes under the couch. A basket full of puppets, dolls, and dress-up items can facilitate interaction at multiple levels within the family.

As with younger children, action needs to replace talk during some of the therapeutic encounters. Sessions can be broken up into sections where the child is "excused" from the therapy (although still in the room) while the therapist talks with parents directly. Therapists must be sure to edit any information that would be inappropriate for the child to overhear. The child can then be reengaged toward the end of the session for a summary of what the family might do during the week to continue improvement. After a session, stickers or other small items to reward the child's participation might encourage involvement in the future.

Besides working with the family itself, therapists must be mindful of what other "system players" need to be involved for therapy to proceed effectively. For example, since at this stage therapy is often initiated due to school concerns, contact with a teacher or other school personnel can significantly enhance work in the family therapy session. Minuchin, Montalvo, Guerney, Rosman, and Schumer (1967) recognize that demands from multiple systems (family, child, and school) often create problems, rather than the child being the problem.

Active information gathering from the school, childcare, or sports or religious organizations with which the family is involved can be useful in shaping appropriate interventions. Whether the presenting problem occurs only in one setting or across multiple settings helps the therapist to orient his or her approach with the family. The following case demonstrates how interventions involving outside settings are both important and beneficial.

Brittany was a 12-year-old girl enrolled in the seventh grade. She was brought to therapy by her parents because she was having problems in school. She had done well in elementary school, achieving mostly As and Bs. After entering junior high school she hadn't performed well academically, getting Cs and Ds at the end of the first semester. She complained that she didn't like most of her teachers. She would do most of her homework but often "forgot" to turn it in. The parents reported no problems at home. She did most of her chores when she was asked and enjoyed playing softball and playing piano.

Brittany was a soft-spoken, bright, and articulate girl who felt "badly" about her school performance. She blamed most of the problem on a couple of her teachers who, she said, "don't like me and are boring." She often felt intimidated by the teachers and the school environment. She found going to different classes and having lots of teachers to be disruptive and chaotic. She was also struggling with making new friends and was feeling that she didn't fit in. Her response to feeling overwhelmed by the new school environment was to withdraw. She became afraid of failing, so decided not to turn in her homework. The more she got behind in her classes the more her feelings of failure and futility increased.

The parents responded that they were "concerned, frustrated, and helpless" about Brittany's school problems. The father was often out of town because of his work and he didn't have enough contact with Brittany to "truly understand the problems." The mother was frustrated in her attempts to help Brittany. She had tried to help the girl with her homework, but they would end up quarreling. She felt that Brittany wasn't interested in talking about school and would either withdraw or become defensive. Brittany's mother had contacted the school counselor but felt that the counselor was of little help. The counselor suggested that Brittany might need a tutor and that her test scores indicated that Brittany was "full of potential and easily capable of doing the work."

The therapist began working with the family, although the father's attendance was sporadic due to his work commitments. Brittany and her mother had a fairly close relationship. They spent a fair amount of time together and genuinely enjoyed each other's company. They shared interests in music and sports, and played tennis together. Their primary difficulty revolved around Brittany's school problems and an inability to communicate without arguing about school.

Brittany was having considerable difficulty in making the adjustment from the stable elementary school environment to the fluctuating schedule at the junior high school. She felt insecure and overwhelmed by the constant changes in her classes, the lack of individual attention, and the sheer number of students. The therapist contacted the school counselor in an effort to increase the school's interest in Brittany, and to obtain more structure and stability for her. The counselor said the school would cooperate in providing weekly progress reports on Brittany's work. The counselor also agreed to provide a student mentor for Brittany. The mentor would be an eighth-grader who could help tutor Brittany and help familiarize her with the school. The mother was encouraged to contact several of Brittany's teachers and coordinate their efforts in determining whether Brittany turned in her homework.

Brittany responded very positively to the structure and interest she was given. Her adjustment to the new school was slower than that of most students and she needed some special attention. The therapist was able to intervene to work as a liaison between the school and the family and to support positive solutions to Brittany's adjustment.

Families with Adolescents

The primary emotional task for families at this stage is increasing the family's boundary permeability to allow for children's growing independence. Flexibility may or may not be characteristic of the family throughout its history. Often this stage also signals a time in which the growing frailties of grandparents must be considered.

Second only to the life cycle period with young children, this stage is associated with a high number of divorces. One reason is the convergence of many powerful and sometimes competing needs of family members. First, the adolescent must be permitted to move in and out of the family system more fluidly. Friendships and relationships outside the family take on growing significance and the family sometimes becomes secondary in the young person's life. When family values conflict with the teenager's behavioral choices, the family might over- or underrespond. In either case, family therapy can enhance positive adaptation to this stage.

Issues besides adolescence are present at this stage—midlife concerns for parents often come to the fore. Regrets, missed opportunities, possibilities for beginning new dreams, reassessing the quality of the marital relationship, all add to the challenging mix. Further, stresses from taking care of older parents emerge. Such caretaking consumes time and financial resources. Adults in these families often term themselves "caught in the middle" between the financial and emotional needs of their older and younger members. The following case illustrates the interplay between difficulties around adolescence and midlife issues:

The C family was having difficulty with their youngest child, 15-year-old Derrick, who hadn't been coming home at night, was doing poorly at school, and had been caught with marijuana on several occasions. Derrick was a star football player on his high school team. He was a bright, likable, and outgoing young man who appeared self-assured. He came from a family of four children, in which the other three were out of the home—two in college and one in the navy. This was a middle-class, African American family that had come to a point in its development in which everyone seemed to be going off in separate directions.

Derrick's mother was a 54-year-old woman who had worked hard most of her life at her civil service job while raising her four children. She was very involved in her church, and after her parents died she had become the matriarch of her family. She had a younger sister who was a single mother and was trying to raise three children. Mrs. C spent a great deal of her time helping her sister. She also helped out with her husband's printing business. Mr. C was a 57-year-old man who had retired from the navy about 12 years ago. He had worked hard to develop his own business, which had lots of financial problems. Mr. C was rarely at home and spent his time at work or with his friends.

Mr. and Mrs. C were concerned about Derrick's behavior, but both acknowledged that they were tired of raising children. They had worked hard and fulfilled their responsibilities. They were helping all of their children financially and felt burdened by this. They expressed a desire to slow things down and spend some time together, and they had been talking about wanting a less hectic lifestyle. Mr. C wanted to sell his business and move to Arizona. Derrick wasn't sure where he fit into the picture; he felt his parents really didn't care what he did, as long as he stayed out of trouble. He said that he got very little attention from them and "that's okay, they don't really know what I'm doing." Mrs. C expressed a lot of concern and frustration with the situation but didn't know what to do. She said she just didn't have the energy to deal with Derrick.

Derrick's difficulties seemed symptomatic of his confusion over recent changes and his perceived lack of security in the family. There was a considerable difference in needs and priorities between Derrick and his parents. They readily admitted that they couldn't keep up with him. Derrick's difficulties in school, marijuana use, and staying out at night could be seen as a cry for attention from his parents and a request for help. Therapy initially needed to validate each family member's position and use their concern for each other as an effective motivation to effect some change. Normalizing their situation given their different needs and developmental stages was also important.

Transformations

Precisely when adolescence begins and ends is open to debate. But one of the most clearly pronounced signs of its beginning is the development of the physical capacity to procreate. Secondary sex characteristics overtly signal this transition, and social definitions become more sexually oriented. Children can grasp ideas and concepts beyond their own concrete experience, that is, they are able to think more abstractly, although this capacity is measured in different ways across cultures. On the social-emotional front, teenagers struggle with self-definition. They "try on" roles, like trying on jeans at a department store, in order to find the right fit. Without this process, individuals become confused about who they are in life. Parental overreaction to this natural developmental stage can stigmatize a child as "a problem" and lead the adolescent to retreat from family connections. Underreaction, too, can hinder this stage, leaving nonfamily agencies such as the school or police to provide the only limit setting for the adolescent.

Therapists attempt to balance the family need for maintaining structure with the transformational needs of launching an adolescent member. This balance is aided, in part, when the therapist manages the IP label appropriately, creates a metaphor or ritual to capture the family's evolution, and is flexible in responding to the idiosyncrasies of the family.

For example, a 17-year-old adolescent and his family came to therapy with the presenting problem of his drug use. The boy had been experimenting with various drugs and his schoolwork had declined. The family focused on the son's problems so intently that everything seemed to revolve around him—who or who did not do the chores, fights between siblings, and conflict between the parents. The therapist created a family sculpt exercise in order to show the family its developmental dilemma. She first asked the client to sit in a chair in the middle of the therapy room and asked each family member to stand in emotional proximity to him. A closely connected "huddle" resulted. She then removed the son from the middle and stated that she was going to work with him on his issues, and asked the rest of the family to stand where they would like to be in the family. Confusion resulted. The family members looked lost, unable to glimpse a vision of life without the IP's presence. Debriefing following the session evoked important and unacknowledged emotions from various family members about the "positive" function the client served for the family. The family had become developmentally stuck and unable to move forward because of their fears of separateness and individuality.

Most commonly, teenagers are brought to therapy to be "fixed" by the therapist. Although the rest of the family members acknowledge, at some level, that they impact the adolescent, often the focus is "teen versus the family system." Family therapists do well to bring up the complexities of this developmental stage with the family. Psychoeducation helps the family broaden its frame of reference and normalizes the anxiety for everyone. "How are we going to help this child become an adult?" is a useful question to be presented to the entire family. Probing how the parents went through this stage can elicit normalizing information not discussed by the family previously. Having parents describe what their own parents did well or poorly during this stage provokes some systemic reflection.

The therapist should keep in mind, however, that the family isn't the only important concern during this stage. If an adolescent has been displaying addictive patterns, relationships outside of the family might be affecting the teen, and may involve drug use or sexual activity. When the therapist thinks about multiple systems rather than family systems alone, other factors are seen as important to therapeutic work. Referral to a chemical dependency program or inviting friends into therapy might be helpful in managing these important influences. Creatively engaging people from within and without the family to understand the presenting problem assists in solid clinical treatment.

Most civilizations have heralded the passage from childhood to adulthood. Western culture, however, is generally bereft of meaningful ways to mark this transition. Perhaps the most significant ritual for teens in the United States is acquiring a driver's license. Therapists have found that bringing a ritual into the therapeutic process can assist in creating second-order change (Imber-Black, 1988). Rituals can awaken family members to respond in new ways. One therapist assigned a family the task of creating a "birthday ritual" for each quarter-, half-, and full-year birthday beginning at age 15 and ending at age 18. Using these "birthdays" as points for change, the family negotiated one new privilege for their daughter and one new responsibility. The parents and teenager talked about ways in which they needed to both offer more adulthood status and she needed to show more adulthood behavior. Issues such as curfew, driving, chores, and allowance were "ritually" discussed on these dates until a mutual agreement was found. A celebration of adulthood was prescribed for her 18th birthday.

As so often happens, therapists and clients are challenged by the same things during therapy. Families with adolescents need to be flexible, and so does the therapist. Therapists encounter teenagers who may angrily sulk during most sessions and then suddenly rage at everyone. Parents of teenagers may present as flexible, yet undermine any new suggestions developed during therapy.

Therapists need to keep in mind their "window of opportunity" to influence a family positively. Settling into a long-term therapy posture probably won't fit the needs of the family. Even a weekly therapy schedule might need to be reevaluated. Working with various subsystems of the family, as with very young children, can be quite valuable. Encouraging adolescents to do reverse role plays (in which the teen plays the parent) or to write poems and letters to express their feelings to the family might enhance therapy, too.

Maintaining a balance between structural expectations (regarding physical safety or time together) and flexibility around the presenting concerns helps develop a strong therapeutic alliance and will model to the family what they need to be doing in their home as well.

Launching Children and Later Life

Issues around launching children and experiencing later life become more prominent as economic instability and life expectancy increase. Families are challenged to accept multiple comings and goings in the family system's membership. In-laws, grandchildren, returning divorced children, aging parents, and death must be accommodated during this life stage. Couples often shift into a dyadic relationship for the first time in life, and are challenged to create a non-child-oriented relationship. Adolescents grow into adults who have their own children, and relationships with them shift from parent–child to adult–adult connections. Illness, retirement, or disability challenge the family's resources at many turns. Additions and losses pervade the emotional terrain.

Family therapists can act as consultants during this stage. Clients often request a few brief sessions to "sort out what to do next": "Shall I kick my 27-year-old cocaine-addicted son out of my home?" "Shall we bring Grandma in to live with us after her stroke?" "I thought I was going to have time to travel with my husband, but now we're helping to raise my grandchildren while my daughter works—I'm not sure I want this, but I feel guilty saying that."

We are in changing societal times with few clear directives on how to handle these complex and emotionally charged issues. Each family needs to redefine itself in response to its unique set of beliefs, structural framework, and emotional capacity.

Physically, most people peak in strength and agility during this stage and then move toward progressive deterioration. Particularly for those who have defined themselves in physical terms (attractive, athletic), this stage requires new adjustment around one's self-concept.

Ultimately, personal and relational functioning is connected to the extent of physiological decline. In a culture that encourages independence and celebrates youth, attention to physical decline becomes pronounced in later years. Along with physical concerns, cognitive abilities may be affected by aging. Although people maintain a high ability to continue to learn, new information may be processed more slowly. Memory and reaction time can be impaired, and a small but significant number of people are seriously impacted by dementia and

Alzheimer's disease. Caretaking by family members continues to be the key resource for those affected by aging difficulties.

Social-emotional needs of those being launched from a family include the development of intimate relationships and some sort of generativity in the world. Friends and lovers must be found and relationships established. Often individuals seek therapy when limited in this important developmental domain. Being able to use one's gifts, abilities, and interests for the benefit of self and others takes on a prominent focus. Having at least some degree of financial independence from one's family seems to be a part of the process. If these needs aren't met, people experience isolation and stagnation. Often it is in midlife that these concerns are recycled and reviewed once again, although losing one's job or suffering a business failure elicits reassessment, too.

Later in life, social-emotional needs involve reviewing one's life choices and evaluating whether one feels integrated regarding what has been accomplished. Peer relationships continue to be a vital connection to good health, although family contacts are important in emergencies. Solid friendships in later years promote well-being at many levels. Gender concerns reemerge as one reviews personal and professional connections. Some men in our culture feel too separated from family connections, while women ponder if they could have been something more than what they were. In either case, a life review in connection with continuing family and friendship ties enhances relationships between all members.

Helping clients access resources and deal with grief are important skills a therapist can apply when working with families in launching and later-life stages. Although useful throughout the lifespan, knowledge of community and extended family resources can be critical during these periods. The therapist can encourage clients to use some of their own resources and use community resources in achieving positive adjustment for the entire family. Financial, emotional, and practical information can be provided that helps ease some of the strains of this stage. Two cases illustrate these points.

John, age 20, began to have difficulties while away at college. A history major, he had dreams of becoming a lawyer after he finished college. He began drinking heavily during his junior year, and his friends reported to his family that he was acting a bit odd at times. On one occasion, he jumped down a long flight of stairs screaming that the "monkeys were trying to bite me." Hospitalization for a broken ankle and for his first schizophrenic episode followed. John took a leave of absence from college, never to return. When he went home, however, his family found it difficult to cope with him.

Martha, age 78, lived alone after the death of her husband 10 years previously. She lived independently, enjoyed her friends, and gardened and walked each day. One day, her daughter called her several times and did not reach her—an unusual experience. A friend was asked to check on her, and she found Martha unconscious on the floor. Taken to the hospital immediately, Martha was diagnosed with a small cerebral hemorrhage that disabled her permanently. She was unable to walk independently, and thus could no longer live alone or take care of herself. The family faced the decision of what to do next.

In each of these two cases, a family therapist may be included in the decision-making process. The therapist will need to assess the resources of the family as well as the values they hold regarding care for their ill relatives, and may encourage them to broaden their support to include extended family and friends. Also, he or she may be able to access important community resources for the family and assist them in learning to network. Medical specialists, funding sources, self-help and support groups, board and care homes, transitional housing options, respite care, and practical nursing can be invaluable resources for the family.

Therapists who have difficulty managing grief issues would not be well suited for work with families in these stages of the life cycle. Developmentally, the family needs to go through various processes in order to manage either the symbolic or actual death of its members. These include the following:

1. Shared acknowledgment of the death or loss—someone is "gone."
2. Shared expressions of the range of emotions—allow for variations.
3. Reorganization of the family system to accommodate loss—the practical ability for the family to continue to function.
4. Reinvestment into a future life direction without the loved one—finding new ways to continue a meaningful life.

Therapists must assess whether the family has gone through each of these stages and can facilitate any unfinished dimensions of the grieving.

VARIATIONS IN FAMILY DEVELOPMENT

Of course, the stages of the family life cycle described above address just part of a family's development over time. In addition to the transitions associated with family members joining or leaving a system, families encounter many other unpredictable transitions over time, such as job loss, geographical relocation and migration, serious illness, divorce, and many other challenges that have a major impact on family life. The following sections describe family adjustment to divorce and explore two variations in family structure: single-parent families and stepfamilies.

Divorce

Family adjustment to divorce comprises additional stages in the family life cycle—stages that are almost normative in a society where divorce is so common. Stress occurs at predictable times for divorcing families, and the response to the stress influences how members adjust to shifting family compositions. Family therapists need to keep in mind that emotional cutoffs often hinder adjustment and that, even though there are exceptions, having an ongoing relationship between parents and children is usually the best way to proceed.

The family therapy literature provides numerous examples of how divorcing families go through predictable stages (Ahrons & Rodgers, 1987; Everett & Volgy, 1991; Kaslow, 2000). Most of the stage models share a general framework, which includes (1) predivorce issues, such as feelings of ambivalence; (2) the decision to divorce; and (3) postdivorce adjustment, restructuring, and, in many cases, remarriage (Livingston & Bowen, 2006). For example, Ahrons and Rodgers found divorcing families go through the following stages, although not necessarily in sequential order:

1. Decision to divorce, usually by one member before the other
2. Family system is told about the impending divorce
3. Actual physical separation
4. System reorganization
5. System stabilization into a new form

Most researchers indicate that it takes 2–3 years to go through these phases. Successful postdivorce families may often look like the following:

Single parent
- Maintains parental contact with ex-spouse.
- Supports contact of children with ex-spouse and his or her family.
- Rebuilds own social network.

Noncustodial parent

- Maintains parental contact and supports custodial parent's relationship with children.
- Establishes effective parenting relationship with children.
- Rebuilds own social network.

However, research also indicates that only about half of divorcing families are able to develop cooperative coparenting arrangements. The other half of divorced parents continue to fight with their former spouse over the children or neglect this continuing aspect of their relationship. Family therapists often see the emotional fallout on the children from these negative experiences.

Divorce almost always involves some level of conflict. The research affirms again and again that children exposed to continuing parental conflict are negatively affected. Individuals and families will not be able to move beyond their presenting problems unless they can manage conflict constructively. Therapists must advise and set limits on the amount of conflict permitted within the family (Margulies, 2007).

In addition, therapists must determine how able a family is to operate in a coparenting relationship. When parents are unable to cooperate for the sake of their children, therapists must consider how to define relationships between parents and children separately. Complete cutoff with a parent might occur, but should not be an acceptable solution for the family. Effective coparenting by coparents who can cooperate and continued contact with noncustodial parents, typically fathers, will play a significant role in helping children adjust to divorce (Ahrons, 2007).

Therapists should guard against colluding with particular family members because doing so can close off relationships that might be therapeutic. For example, a mother might say that her ex-husband has "no interest" in their difficult teenage daughter. If you contact the father, however, you may find he does have an interest and can assist the family and support his ex-wife in parenting the teen. Each case regarding connections with noncustodial parents needs to be considered carefully.

Often extended family—aunts, uncles, grandparents, and cousins—had significant relationships severed as a result of divorce. These relatives can often function as family resources during difficult transitional stages. Therapists should ask about these people and encourage contact when appropriate.

When working with families experiencing divorce, it's important to remind family members that it takes time and patience to negotiate these stages successfully. Some don't manage well because of the continuing battles between family members. Noticing and encouraging successful developmental steps and normalizing struggles will help families use their resources to the fullest.

Mediation and Child Custody Evaluation

Family therapists have become an important resource for the legal system in determining the separating and postdivorce world of the family. Many states require families to work with family court mediators, a large number of whom have family therapy training, to assist a family in negotiating divorce and custody settlements. Mediators have helped to relieve our overburdened court system in many states. Specialized training allows mediators to become an important link between the legal and family systems.

Most states' legal systems have moved from the "tender years doctrine" of generally awarding mothers custody to a "best interests of the child" standard. The Uniform Marriage and Divorce Act (National Conference of Commissioners on Uniform State Laws, 1970) offers these guidelines in Section 402:

> The court shall determine custody in accordance with the best interest of the child. The court shall consider all relevant factors, including:
>
> 1. the wishes of the child's parent or parents as to his custody;
> 2. the wishes of the child as to his custodian;
> 3. the interaction and interrelationship of the child with his parent or parents, his siblings, and any other person who may significantly affect the child's best interest;
> 4. the child's adjustment to his home, school, and community; and
> 5. the mental and physical health of all individuals involved.
>
> The court shall not consider conduct of a proposed custodian that does not affect his relationship to the child.

Judges often rely on the advice of experts to determine the "best interests" standard; this relational information can be obtained from a family therapist's observations and opinions. Parents as well as the court can seek the services of family therapists for this purpose. Sometimes interns and therapists are surprised to discover the "true" motive for a person seeking therapy after it has been going on for a while— the client requests a letter or report from the therapist to be used in a divorce court or custody proceeding.

Therapists need to be informed about the divorce and custody laws of their state in order to work competently in this arena. If one wants to learn how to do custody evaluations, it is best to be mentored by someone who has done them over several years and is recognized by the court. Therapists need to be aware of the research outcomes regarding high-conflict divorce. Finally, therapists need a clear contract regarding their role in any divorce or custody case. Often, it's best to be hired as an expert to the court rather than be triangulated into serving as an expert for one parent against the other parent. Family therapists have much to contribute to the legal–family interface (Gould & Martindale, 2007).

Single-Parent Families

Whether the result of divorce, death, or a choice to parent alone, single-parent families, usually headed by the mother (U.S. Census Bureau, 2000), share many common challenges that have the potential to go unrecognized in the therapy room. When a child from a single-parent family is presented to you for therapy, you will benefit by identifying and addressing these challenges, most notably the possible challenges of financial stress and the fact that many single-parent families are coping with loss, whether it be the loss of a partner/parent or the loss of a dream about a family's future (Anderson, 2003).

Due to work and family demands, single parents frequently feel overwhelmed and depleted by their varied roles and responsibilities. In addition, children of single parents may carry a greater share of the domestic responsibilities because their sole parent is working outside the home. Because strands of American culture have often been critical of single-family structure, it is common for single parents to live with the guilt of "not being good enough."

Minuchin, Colapinto, and Minuchin (2006) offer a clinical approach to working with single-parent, low-income families that includes structurally defining parental roles when parents, live-in partners, and grandparents have a say about the household's children; encouraging the development of the biological mother's personal resources; and increasing access to social and economic resources. The following case provides a glimpse of what life can be like for clients who are single mothers living in poverty, as well as some appropriate interventions.

Ms. G was a single mother who was raising three children: 7-year-old Elise, 10-year-old Alex, and 13-year-old Gilbert. Ms. G's husband had left the family when Elise was 2 years old, and he had provided no support and had no contact with the children. This family lived in a small two-bedroom apartment. The mother worked long hours cleaning office buildings, and she had little money to pay for anything but the bare essentials. Her long hours made supervision of the children difficult, so she often left Gilbert in charge. This became an increasingly difficult situation because he resented the responsibility and would leave his brother and sister alone for long periods.

Ms. G sought counseling at the recommendation of the school counselor. Gilbert had become a "behavior problem" at school. After entering junior high school a year and a half before, he began cutting classes and showing little interest in his schoolwork. His mother said that he was hanging out with "gang bangers," but she didn't think that Gilbert was involved in a gang. She had tried to get his uncle to spend time with Gilbert but his work schedule made this difficult. Gilbert seemed angry with and disappointed by any authority figures. His grades kept dropping and his teachers had added Saturday school as a steady part of his weekly routine.

Ms. G felt frustrated and helpless in trying to handle Gilbert. She said she was almost ready to give up and concentrate on the younger ones. She couldn't afford to pay for childcare after school and so had begun to send the younger children to the local Boys and Girls Club, but she was afraid of the effects that the older neighborhood children would have on Alex and Elise.

Ms. G had been receiving some help from her mother until they began having difficulties about 2 years earlier. Ms. G had begun dating a man that her mother disliked, and this caused considerable conflict between the two women. The children's grandmother wanted to maintain contact with them but Ms. G's anger and resentment caused her to severely limit their visits.

Ms. G's lack of financial resources and emotional support was quite apparent. The therapist's job was to assist her in making effective use of community resources and in considering family therapy that would include the children, Ms. G, and her mother. Single parents like Ms. G often lack the time and energy to make use of community resources and feel overwhelmed in attempting to fulfill all of their responsibilities. Providing support and identifying outside resources is an essential element in working with this type of case.

While single-parent families often face daunting problems, most of them are competent and successful. Lindblad-Goldberg (1989) has identified successful single-parent families as those in which parents, usually mothers, showed less depression, experienced more control over their lives, displayed more effective executive authority with their children, launched their older children from the household, communicated more effectively, developed close family ties, cognitively highlighted positive life experiences rather than negative ones, and used social networks creatively. When working with single parents or children of single parents, it is imperative that you address their hardships and highlight their strengths and resilience.

Stepfamilies

In the aftermath of divorce and death, parents often remarry and form stepfamilies. Unlike first marriages with no children, stepfamilies face the daunting task of merging two families with different beliefs, traditions, and practices; they also must sort out a variety of roles and responsibilities. For example, who will discipline the children and what methods of discipline will be used? Although all families confront this question, stepfamilies must cope with many unique issues, such as family loyalties (will children accept the new stepparent?) and role ambiguity (what parenting responsibilities does a stepparent want or expect?).

Papernow (1993) described seven stages that stepfamilies go through: (1) Fantasy—adults have expectations of instant love in a ready-made family; (2) Immersion—a sense of discomfort and evidence of tension and conflict; (3) Awareness—members getting to know themselves and each other in the new system; (4) Mobilization—coping with struggles over differences while maintaining momentum from earlier stages; (5) Action—strengthening of the couple's relationship and greater cohesion among new family members; (6) Contact—stepparent–stepchild relationship becomes closer and more authentic and some stability has been achieved; and (7) Resolution—members experience their step relationships as reliable and nourishing. It can take stepfamilies many years to work through these stages. Sharing this information with stepfamilies can help validate and normalize their experiences. Validation and normalization helps the family see you as someone who understands the unique challenges of stepfamilies, and it has been shown to be a helpful intervention for stepfamilies (Pasley, Rhoden, Visher, & Visher, 1996).

Although it's rare for a client to label a problem as a "stepfamily problem" and whole stepfamilies rarely arrive at a therapist's office for the first appointment, stepfamily dynamics are a common, important undercurrent that you need to address. Of particular importance are the quality of the couple's relationship, stepparent–stepchild relationships, and, in the case of divorce, the level of cooperation between former spouses in their roles as coparents. The following case illustrates some of the problems encountered by stepfamilies.

Mr. and Mrs. A presented with arguing and disagreements over raising their two boys. They were a recently married couple, and each spouse had an 11-year-old boy. Most of the couple's other disagreements seemed to be resolvable, but discussions involving the boys would quickly escalate, with Mr. A becoming very angry and Mrs. A crying and feeling attacked and hopeless. Each partner accused the other of being overly protective of his or her own child. The husband's response to the conflict was to become openly angry, raise his voice, and become opinionated and a bit self-righteous. The wife would cry, withdraw, and say that she had never been talked to like this before. Both agreed that if this problem was not resolved they could not stay married. Mr. A threatened to leave if his wife wouldn't change. There was no indication of physical violence and very little alcohol use.

The husband was a 42-year-old insurance adjuster, retired navy officer, and Vietnam veteran. He was 21 years old when he married for the first time. That marriage lasted for 3 years, and he was not sure why it ended. His son was born during his second marriage, which lasted 6 years. That relationship ended because his wife started seeing other men. He described his ex-wife as irresponsible and childlike. His son had occasional contact with her. Mr. A's family of origin was described as a "good learning experience." His father was a career marine officer and his mother was a homemaker. His parents' marriage was described as tumultuous. They divorced when he was 14.

Mr. A was a very committed and concerned father who was very close to his son. He was a proud man who spoke directly and expressed his opinions freely. He was involved with his son in sports and his schoolwork, and they liked to travel together. His son was a good student, well mannered, and an excellent athlete.

Mrs. A was a 40-year-old physical therapist. She had been married for 12 years; her husband had died abruptly of a heart attack about 3 years earlier. He was 40 years old at the time. She cared for him very much and described him as "sensitive, caring, easy to get along with, but a bit boring." She came from a very religious, conservative, stable family environment. Her parents were happily married and had been supportive throughout her marriage and since the death of her husband. She described herself as easygoing, sensitive, and emotional. She was very close to her son and felt bad that he had lost his father. Her son was bright, conservative, and did well in school. He was not particularly good at sports but excelled in math, science, and computers.

Mr. A had some negative feelings about therapy. He went with his ex-wife and had found it of little value. Mrs. A was afraid that without help they would likely get a divorce because of the fights and Mr. A's primary allegiance to his son. Mrs. A said, "We just can't agree about anything the boys do, and the smallest thing turns into a major battle every time."

This case demonstrates that stepfamilies do not, and cannot, come together as biological families do. The newly married (or committed) couple must find ways to protect their developing relationship (Visher & Visher, 1988, 1996). Children fare better and remarriage is stronger when spouses focus on establishing a strong, supportive, and positive marriage (Hetherington & Stanley-Hagan, 2002). The new partners also need to figure out how to form an effective parenting team. Allegiances between a biological parent and child remain strong, and in the early going, need to be protected. In general, stepparents should tread lightly but consistently in their attempts to connect with their stepchildren. Rushing in as a disciplinarian, expecting instant love, trying to replace the biological parent, or acting as the biological parent's equal is rarely well received. Children tend to reject stepparents who discipline and try to control them early on (Ganong, Coleman, Fine, & Martin, 1999). The stepparent who is patient and supportive and persists in his or her efforts to achieve closeness is more likely to receive affection from stepchildren (Bray & Kelly, 1998).

CONCLUSION

In this chapter, we have reviewed information on the predictable and unpredictable changes in the lives of families with children. Knowledge of a family's lifespan and the presenting problems associated with each developmental stage and transition assists us in providing solid clinical work. Family therapists need to recognize their strengths and limitations when assisting families through their growing pains. At a time when social transitions are complex and abundant, it is impossible to provide a single model of family that fits every family. Rather, we walk alongside families to help them invent a new form of family structure that will work for them.

CHAPTER 8

Working with Couples

M ary is a 29-year-old Caucasian woman who has been recovering from alcoholism for the past year. Bob is a 32-year-old Caucasian male who is also recovering from alcoholism. Bob is being treated for depression by a psychiatrist who is prescribing Lexapro for him. Mary has been to two individual therapists through her health maintenance organization but feels dissatisfied with them because they don't really understand "the disease" of alcoholism.

This couple has been living together for the past 6 years. They have separated several times during that period. They were married 1 year ago. Bob says that he is increasingly unhappy in the marriage and has decided that he wants a separation. Mary has said that she "can't stand the thought of being without him" and wants to keep the relationship together. She reports "always feeling insecure" and doubting herself. She feels very confused by Bob's "double messages" because he says he wants a divorce but continues to act friendly and interested in Mary. He invites her to do things with him and desires to be with her sexually. He also tells Mary that he doesn't love her anymore. They argue and bicker about lots of little things but seem able to discuss important concerns. Still, many conflicts go unresolved.

Mary is requesting couple therapy to "try to either resolve these issues or get some closure." Bob is reluctant to go to therapy but has indicated that he will try it for one or two visits. They saw a couple therapist previously but didn't continue, as Mary felt that the therapist sided with Bob and didn't really understand the situation.

This case presents a complex web of symptoms and concerns. The individual issues include the alcoholism, Bob's depression, and Mary's low self-esteem. The couple's issues include their confusion about whether to stay together, their inability to resolve conflict, and their poor communication. The case is complicated by their previous unsatisfactory attempt at therapy. How does a therapist understand and work with such a couple?

This chapter focuses on couples who seek help for their continuing relationship. We explain the key principles that beginning (and probably all) therapists need to follow to do effective couple therapy. We then move to special topics in couple therapy and suggest ways to understand and deal with them.

KEYS TO PROVIDING SOLID COUPLE THERAPY

What makes a good couple therapist? There are some unique aspects of doing couple therapy that can make the therapist's job difficult. Knowing about some of these and, more importantly, anticipating them can ease some of the difficulty. Implementing the key principles described below will increase the likelihood that couple work will be successful.

Key Number 1: Joining with the Couple System

Effective couple therapists must have the ability to manage a three-person relationship. Managing this three-person relationship, however, can present a challenge for beginning therapists. A new intern, in commenting about her first couple session, said, "I felt beat up, totally stuck in the middle. Anytime I tried to listen to the husband, the wife interrupted and told me her version. I didn't know what to do." The therapist literally becomes the emotional and relational hub for the couple's interactions, and can provide the foundation for solid couple work depending on how well he or she works with a triangle, or three-person relationship. Therapists can connect to the couple in several ways, as shown in Figure 8.1.

Creating an Empathic Connection with Each Partner

In the first diagram (Figure 8.1A), the therapist attempts to connect empathically with each person. For example, he or she might ask at the beginning of the first session, "What brings you in today and how might you want me to help?" With this, one partner might say, "I'm not happy in my marriage and I haven't been for a long time. I don't know what to do. I've tried but nothing seems to work." The therapist might empathically respond, "So you're sad and frustrated with the way your marriage is right now and you're confused about what to do next." The

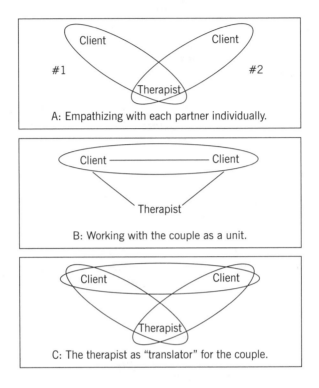

FIGURE 8.1. Therapeutic triangles.

client responds, "Yes, that's it." When the therapist builds the relationship with each person during the first session, then each one usually experiences a beginning bond and trust with the therapist and will want to continue in therapy.

It's important to remember that when the therapist takes an individually empathic position, it impacts the triadic relationship. The partner who is not being attended to feels "left out" for a moment. Often the unattended person will interrupt the process to receive attention or to "correct" the point stated by the partner. If the therapist allows this interruption to occur repeatedly without taking charge of the interactions, he or she will begin to feel bumped back and forth between the two individuals, much like a tennis ball between two players. It's wise for the therapist to direct this interaction, to tell the couple that each of them will get their turn, and to emphasize that it's important for the therapist to understand each person's concerns.

Unfortunately, beginning therapists often get stuck at this stage. They know how to connect with each partner, in a sense to begin individual therapy with each, but don't know where to go next. Instead of managing the entire triangle, the therapist listens only to each partner individually during the session. Often the tension between the couple heightens and the interaction becomes more conflicted. Without knowing how to manage the case triadically, the therapist might even recommend each person be seen separately. Although this is useful at times, most often couple work needs to be done with both partners present. Separating the couple mostly helps the therapist's anxiety, not the couple's need to work on things together. In order to be effective, the therapist must be able to move fluidly to other positions.

Working with the Couple as a Unit

An alternative approach to working with the couple is to make the couple's relationship the focus rather than each person (Figure 8.1B). Rather than focus on the personal therapist–client relationship, the therapist takes a position of orchestrating new behaviors between the couple. Much of traditional couple therapy, especially any with psycho-educational or "skill training" components, takes this triadic stance. Skills and positive interactional experiences are needed to create and maintain a new couple system.

For example, a couple comes to therapy presenting with fights over parenting and money. The therapist determines several strengths in their relationship and decides to begin therapy with a solution-focused therapy approach. The therapist begins to identify when they "don't fight" and to describe these interactions in detail. She also explores and "rates" when their fights are "less destructive" to their relationship. She encourages the couple to notice when they are doing "not fighting" behaviors and "less destructive" fighting styles. After several weeks, the couple reports "less intense" fighting around money and parenting. They also identify that spending weekly "fun time" together sets a better tone in their relationship to discuss problematic issues surrounding money. In this case, the therapist focuses on developing new relationship patterns that address the couple's presenting problems. Individual experiences are less of a focus; the therapist is more goal directed and works with the couple as a unit.

When a beginning therapist is unsure of how to proceed when doing work with a couple or when a couple negatively escalates their interaction, the therapist can interrupt the process by restating the powerful assumption of this triadic position; for example, "What we're trying to do here is create a new kind of relationship where both of your concerns and needs can be honored. Rather than living together as opponents, let's work on being on the same team." Another comment from this perspective might be "We all know that partnering is hard work. In many ways, you've never been 'married' on this issue and this is the first time you're trying to find a really useful way to work it out."

These kinds of comments often lessen the tension between the couple since both are joined in wanting to make the relationship work. If this doesn't calm them, it may mean that at least one person has already emotionally left the relationship and has given up attempting to be a partner (Gottman & Notarius, 2000). Alternatively, it might indicate the therapist's need to return to the previously discussed "empathic" position with respect to one of the partners. In such a case, the therapist should attend to and possibly reengage the more disengaged partner.

The Therapist as "Translator" for the Couple

A final triadic position the therapist can take to manage couple therapy effectively is that of an interpreter or translator (Figure 8.1C). In this focus, the therapist functions as one who understands that each partner's behaviors, perceptions, and experiences influence the couple's functioning. The therapist creates new ways for the couple to understand each other, often taking a mediating or reframing position. For example, couples commonly battle with each other because each person is trying to re-create his or her family of origin in the new relationship. Often both partners want to get back to their own way of understanding their cultural and familial ways of doing things.

What the therapist needs to keep in mind is that the couple is in the process of creating a "new system" of relating with each other. Interactions that respect some combination of each person's history and values can help to create this new system. Without this new-system perspective, the couple continues to fight. The therapist can facilitate the creation of the new system by helping each partner better understand where their mate is coming from.

Basic to being a "translator" for the couple is an understanding that requires each person to be validated as "different" in some way. These differences will either promote a healthy, differentiated system or will disintegrate into a power play wherein each partner wants to win control of the relationship. The therapist, rather than taking sides, promotes a relationship based on the unit of the couple rather than on each person individually. The therapist simultaneously translates and verbalizes how each partner brings into the relationship different ways of being and doing.

For example, a young couple comes in with complaints about how they are spending their money. One partner came from a structured family where money was carefully accounted for, while the other partner's family allowed all members to spend as they wished. Each partner argues for his or her own "right way" to oversee the family budget and criticizes the other for being either tight or irresponsible. The therapist can first acknowledge the strengths and possible liabilities of each person's family of origin lessons about money. Then he or she might reframe the couple's battle as "very healthy—each person has a different expertise that can benefit the relationship and both need to be heard." Then the therapist can wonder out loud if the couple might find a way to embrace each other's expertise, and, in so doing, strengthen the marriage. In this way the therapist first translates, then mediates, for the couple.

Key Number 2: Building a Commitment to Therapy

Therapy is more likely to be successful if both partners are committed to the relationship. Unfortunately, one of the frequent challenges facing couple therapists is that one or both individuals may be ambivalent about continuing the relationship. Often one partner will present as wanting to save the marriage, while the other is doubtful it can be saved and is seriously thinking of leaving. Angelica came to therapy very distraught that her husband had left her and said that he wanted a divorce. He agreed to come for a few sessions to see if there was a chance to save their marriage. Her hope was reconciliation and she said, "I will do anything to get him back." The ambivalence presented by one partner has been cited as the primary obstacle in working with separating and divorcing couples (Gurman, 2002). Obviously, the greater the difference in a couple's motivation and desire to repair the relationship, the more likely it is that the issues cannot be resolved.

Even if individuals are highly ambivalent about continuing the relationship, it may be possible to build a commitment to therapy. One way to do this is to initially do a marital or relationship evaluation. Typically the therapist contracts to do the evaluation with the couple for a limited number of sessions. The evaluation is framed as a way of better understanding why the relationship is not working. To the ambivalent partner, you can suggest that gaining this understanding is important even if the couple separates or divorces. Otherwise, individuals are at risk for making similar mistakes in future relationships. To the committed partner, you can say that understanding why the relationship is struggling may give insight into how it might be fixed.

Using the metaphor of a home inspector for the evaluation resonates with many couples. Much like a house inspector does for potential home buyers, you will carefully examine the relationship to determine what elements of the relationship need to be fixed, as well as things that seem to be working well. After the evaluation has been completed and presented to the couple, each partner can decide if they want to invest in making the necessary changes to save the relationship. The goal of the evaluation is to give couples new insights into their dynamics, rather than simply list all the problems that exist. The evaluation should also include the strengths that you observe in the relationship. Sometimes offering new insights gives the ambivalent partner some hope that the relationship may be salvageable.

When working with issues of commitment, it is important that you leave the decision up to the client as to whether to continue the relationship. You need to be careful not to push the ambivalent partner to commit to the relationship, or you may create resistance. Conversely, you should not tell an individual to leave a relationship because the problems seem so severe. If you feel that a relationship is unhealthy, then you should clearly state your concerns and what steps the individuals need to take in order to make the relationship healthy.

You can also build a commitment to therapy if you can identify goals for each individual that provide a win–win scenario. In the win–win scenario, the individual will benefit from working on the goals regardless of whether the relationship succeeds or ends. In one marital case, the husband was pursuing his wife for greater connection or closeness. His wife, however, felt smothered by his pursuit. The more he pursued, the more she distanced. The therapist pointed out this dynamic, and suggested that if he continued to pursue her, then he would push her out of the marriage. Thus, the husband was encouraged to examine his dependency needs, which seemed to drive his pursuing behavior. Doing so put the husband in a win–win situation. Working on his dependency issues could help him reduce his pursuing, and perhaps save his marriage by interrupting the couple's vicious cycle. However, if his wife did decide to leave, reducing his dependency needs would make the divorce less painful for him. In a similar manner, the wife was encouraged to explore her ambivalence about intimacy, a pattern that was also evident in her previous relationships. Resolving this issue could potentially help her feel better about the marriage. If she decided to divorce, however, then resolving this issue would still benefit her by helping her avoid replicating this dynamic in future relationships.

Key Number 3: Identifying and Altering Vicious Cycles

In our experience, one of the most powerful predictors as to whether couple therapy is successful is the therapist's ability to identify and alter a couple's negative interactional pattern. These interactional patterns typically take the form of a vicious cycle that the couple repeats over and over, which creates conflict and erodes goodwill within the relationship.

For example, Sandra and Tom, both in their late 40s, presented for couple therapy to work on saving their marriage. Tom, it was recently discovered, had an affair with another woman. The couple reported intense conflict every time they attempted to talk about the affair. The couple appeared stuck in their efforts to move forward. When exploring the conflict over the affair, it was discovered that the couple was caught in a vicious cycle. Sandra would approach Tom with questions about the affair. The questions were an attempt to understand why he had the affair. Tom would begin to retreat from her questioning. When asked why, Tom stated that he wanted to put the affair behind him. He also reported that he was fearful the answers would make his wife even more upset or distressed. Sandra, in contrast, viewed his avoiding her questions as a possible sign that he didn't care about her or that he was protecting the other woman. As a result, his avoidance heightened her distress. The more distressed she became, however, the more convinced Tom became that it was unsafe to talk about the affair. Interrupting this cycle helped the couple begin to feel better about the relationship and got them back on the road to recovery.

The ability to identify and alter negative interactional patterns or vicious cycles is an important skill that family therapists need (see Chapter 6). In many cases, you will be able to directly observe the couple's dynamic in session, particularly if the couple becomes upset when discussing a recent conflict or issue. When anxiety is high in the couple system, couples are likely to fall into their vicious cycle. Circular questioning (see Chapter 6) can often uncover these patterns. For example, you might ask the husband what his wife does next when he complains about her parenting.

When mapping out the cycles, it is important to capture not only what happens behaviorally, but also what each is thinking or feeling that leads them to behave that way. For example, the wife in the example above may feel like a failure or inadequate as a parent when her partner criticizes her, which may lead her to withdraw from parenting. Her withdrawal, in turn, leads her husband to believe that she does not care, which leads him to criticize her more.

It is important to map out the underlying thoughts or feelings since they are often targeted when the therapist attempts to alter the cycle. A cognitively oriented therapist, for example, might challenge the underlying meaning that each attaches to the other's behavior. The therapist might help the husband see that the wife withdraws because of her insecurities about parenting, rather than due to a lack of caring. The husband might then shift his behavior from criticizing his wife to encouraging her in her efforts to parent. Emotionally focused therapists would encourage each party to express his or her primary emotions, which can alter the dynamics (Johnson, 2004). The husband, for example, might be encouraged to express his fear about the children, which his wife's behavior triggers. Through his expressing these primary or softer emotions, she may be able to see beyond his criticisms and be empathetic to his fears regarding the children.

Powerful emotions are often elicited through these patterns, some of which may be connected to one or both of the partners' personal histories. For example, a husband's loud voice may trigger memories of the wife's emotional and physical abuse as a child. The therapist must determine how much historical information is necessary for the partners to work together. Bringing these historical factors into the discussion can sometimes reduce defensiveness on the couple's part, an initial step toward reducing reactivity in the interaction.

In your work with couples, you will notice two commonly encountered patterns, the demand–withdraw cycle and the overfunctioner and underfunctioner cycle. In the demand–withdraw cycle, one partner appears to take the lead more often in working on the couple's relationship. Frequently this is the woman, since women have been socialized to take care of relationship issues more than men. A variation of the demand–withdraw cycle is the pursuer–distancer cycle. In both cases, the pattern develops when one partner initiates and the other responds by backing away. Consider the story of James and Jamie.

Jamie is a 43-year-old Caucasian woman who has been primarily responsible for raising her three children. She works as a teacher and has had to juggle all of her responsibilities since she began to have kids 13 years ago. James is a 45-year-old businessman who works hard at his job, which involves considerable travel. Jamie has felt responsible for running the household, working, and raising the children. She has felt overwhelmed and stressed by all of the tasks and has looked to James for emotional support. They have been married for 15 years. James has been unavailable much of that time. Jamie's requests for support and time are often met with anger from James. He feels that his wife doesn't understand how hard he works, and that when he gets home he wants to be left alone to recover. Jamie's pursuit of time alone with James is often met by his withdrawal and by his working on the computer. He says he wants to do things together, but when he feels ready—not when he feels pushed. The more Jamie pushes James, the more he seems to pull away.

Labeling this interactional sequence for the couple can begin the change process. Celebrating the fact that the distancing partner has come to therapy (which is a nondistancing move) is a reminder of the potential for new patterns to be established. Longitudinal research on marriage shows that some couples manage relationship conflict well, with one partner productively bringing up relationship problems and one who listens and talks, rather than avoiding discussion or shutting down (Gottman, 1999). The individual who brings up problems must approach the partner using a gentle or "soft start-up" in initiating the discussion, while the other remains open to being influenced by him or her.

Another common pattern is the overfunctioner and underfunctioner cycle. The overfunctioner takes on more responsibility in the relationship and is often critical of the other partner for not doing enough. The underfunctioner, in many cases, is happy to let the other partner assume responsibility, reinforcing the overfunctioner's belief that he or she must compensate for the underfunctioner's lack of initiative and responsibility. Interrupting this cycle often requires that the overfunctioner step back, which can create intense anxiety on his or her part (particularly since the underfunctioner may not step in immediately). In addition, you will need to explore possible reasons why the other partner underfunctions. Is it simply because he or she is happy not to have the responsibility, and knows the overfunctioner will do it? Or are there other factors that must be addressed? In some cases, individuals may not feel competent to take the necessary initiative or responsibility, which may or may not be a valid assessment of their abilities. The underfunctioner may also resist doing what the overfunctioner wants unless given the freedom to do it his or her way.

Key Number 4: Moving from Blame to Focus on Self

Couples who present for therapy frequently blame each other for the problems in the marriage or relationship. As long as they remain in this blaming mode, therapy is likely to remain stuck (and frustrating for the therapist). Thus, you will need to get each individual to shift his or her focus away from the partner and focus on what changes he or she needs to make.

Often this can be done in one of several ways. First, it may be possible to identify how the problems in this relationship are similar to those encountered in earlier relationships. This is usually compelling evidence that the individual must have some role in the problem since it repeats itself across a number of different relationships.

Second, identifying the couple's vicious cycle usually illustrates how each partner contributes to the dynamic. Seeing one's part in the cycle can help individuals shift from blaming their partner to focusing on their own thoughts, feelings, or behaviors.

Third, individuals can be reminded that they don't have control over what their partners do. They have control only over themselves. If necessary, you can push this point further by pointing out that they are giving their partner a lot of control over their personal happiness. Partners in oppositional couples may not like this idea, which encourages them to focus more on what they can do themselves to regain a sense of control over their own happiness.

Key Number 5: Strengthening Cohesion and Caring

Couples who come to therapy have often allowed conflict to erode their relationship. Over time, the couple may distance themselves from each other in response to the conflict or to avoid further conflict. Conversely, couples that stop doing pleasurable activities together (e.g., focusing on children) may find that the relationship is more vulnerable to conflict. Regardless of the cause, often an important part of therapy with couples is to strengthen the couple's caring or cohesion.

Building cohesion and caring is often done through prescribing behavioral homework for couples. Getting couples to do pleasurable activities together or go on dates is often a highly effective intervention. Helping couples identify and do more caring behaviors for their partners is also beneficial. Couples who successfully carry through on these homework assignments report greater relationship satisfaction and a greater sense of hope.

Key Number 6: Identifying and Managing Individual Psychopathology

As you will read in the next chapter, therapists must give consideration to how mental illness can impact individuals and families. This is also true for couples, and can complicate treatment. Therefore, when doing couple work, it is important to assess if one or both individuals have any mental illness and/or substance abuse problems, and the extent to which it is impacting the relationship.

In some cases, you may find that the problems in the marriage or relationship are heavily influenced by an undiagnosed mental illness. Mark and Eve, for example, came to therapy after experiencing problems in their 4-year marriage. In the first session, Eve stated that her husband was generally a very kind and considerate man, but around football season he became "Mr. Nasty." She also reported that he would begin to become inactive except for watching a lot of television. Interestingly, the couple also reported that their relationship was great in the summer but would then begin to deteriorate. With further assessment, it was discovered that Mark had a severe case of seasonal affective disorder, which would begin to reappear each fall and go into remission by late spring.

For couples where mental illness is a serious issue, it is important that you encourage individuals (or in some cases, both partners) to get appropriate care or treatment for their disorder. If a mental illness has not been properly managed in the past, then getting appropriate treatment may significantly improve the relationship. One couple reported that conflict in the relationship declined 50–70% after the husband was put on medication for bipolar disorder. A client should be encouraged to learn as much as possible about his or her partner's mental illness. In addition, practicing good self-care should be emphasized, since living with someone with mental illness can be stressful, particularly if the partner is in a caretaking role.

Negative interactional patterns or vicious cycles can arise around mental illness or substance use. Current research has suggested that anxiety disorders may negatively impact the stability and functioning of couples through escalating quarrels, restricting relational behaviors, or decreasing attention to the needs of the nonanxious partner (Snyder, Castellani, & Whisman, 2006). Empirically supported ways to counteract marital dysfunction due to anxiety disorders involve exposure techniques, relaxation techniques, and cognitive restructuring, as suggested by Baucom, Hahlweg, and Kuschel (2003). As an alternative example, a couple may have conflict over one partner's use of alcohol or drugs. The conflict creates tension for the individual using alcohol or drugs, which he or she may try to alleviate by drinking or using again. This, in turn, leads the other partner to attack the individual, creating additional conflict in the relationship. Thus, you may need to concurrently address psychopathology and relational dynamics.

The bidirectional influences of psychopathology and relational dynamics have led to an increased focus on how marital or couple therapy can help treat mental illness or substance abuse. Marital therapy, for example, has been proven to be highly effective in treating depressed spouses (Beach, 2003). Research has found that behavioral couple interventions are increasingly effective in treating, and relieving, symptoms of depression experienced by individuals within a distressed marriage. Effective interventions include an emphasis on behavioral exchange, and on developing communication and problem-solving skills, in addition to cognitive interventions such as practicing a positive frame of mind. Behavioral couples therapy has also been demonstrated to be an effective treatment for substance abuse (Fals-Stewart, Kashdan, O'Farrell, & Birchler, 2002). There is an added benefit of increasing overall marital satisfaction found when practicing behavioral couples therapy, as opposed to practicing therapies that are focused on the individual (Gupta, Coyne, & Beach, 2003).

Key Number 7: Managing Couple Affect

One of the more difficult aspects of doing couple work is that fighting between a couple might escalate, particularly when emotions run high. Couples can bring this high level of conflict into the session, which can be stressful for beginning therapists. Thus, an important part of doing couple work is helping couples manage their affect both within and outside the therapy sessions.

When couples become highly conflictual in the therapy session, you must be comfortable interrupting the interaction. At times, particularly if the couple is "flooded," or in a highly emotional state, this may require that you be quite forceful in getting them to stop. The couple should be encouraged to calm and collect themselves before resuming the discussion. In some cases, it may even be necessary to separate the couple and meet briefly with each of them individually until emotions settle down.

Couples who report that their conflicts escalate should be taught to recognize when one or both is getting flooded. When couples become flooded, they tend to engage in destructive behaviors that damage the relationship. Gottman (1999) has observed that the Four Horsemen—strong predictors of divorce—can invade a relationship when the couple becomes flooded. Individuals who get flooded, for example, may criticize their partner's character or motives rather than make a specific complaint about their partner's behavior. Or, individuals may show contempt, which Gottman believes is particularly corrosive to relationships. Defensiveness and stonewalling are the other two Horsemen. Stonewalling refers to when one partner shuts out the other. Attempts to engage this partner are like speaking to a brick wall. There is also the potential for domestic violence when couples escalate, which should be carefully screened for.

Once a couple is able to recognize that one or both are getting flooded, then someone can ask for a time-out. During the time-out, the couple separates until they have emotionally and physiologically calmed down. Whoever asks for the time-out initially has the responsibility for reinitiating a conversation about the topic. Otherwise, the time-out can be used inappropriately to avoid talking about issues.

Teaching the couple communication skills may help some couples keep from escalating their conflict. The Prevention and Relationship Enhancement Program (PREP; Markman, Stanley, & Blumberg, 2001), for example, teaches couples the "speaker–listener" technique. Using this technique, one partner is the speaker while the other takes the role of listener. After the speaker has had the opportunity to speak as desired, the couple switches roles. The speaker uses skills such as "I" statements to facilitate communication, while the listener uses active or reflective listening to confirm that the message has been correctly understood and received. PREP (Halford, Markman, Kline, & Stanley, 2003), Relationship Enhancement (Cavedo & Guerney, 1999), and Couple Communication (Miller & Sherrard, 1999) are approaches for teaching couples communication and conflict resolution skills that have strong empirical support.

Couples may also need help expressing the softer emotions that are underneath the anger they are expressing. In emotionally focused therapy (Johnson, 2004), a distinction is made between primary and secondary emotions. Primary emotions include sadness, fear, and hurt. Anger is also a primary emotion if it is in response to a boundary violation. However, anger is often a secondary emotion that individuals express rather than the more vulnerable, primary emotions that are underneath. Many individuals, for example, become angry if they become anxious or their partner does something to hurt their feelings. Unfortunately, many individuals have a difficult time dealing with another person's anger, either withdrawing or getting angry in return. In contrast, individuals generally want to comfort those who are sad, fearful, or hurt. Thus, getting clients to express their primary emotions rather than anger may elicit a much different response from their partner. Indeed, getting clients to connect and express their primary emotions can create powerful moments of change in therapy.

SPECIAL TOPICS

Gender, cultural, and societal factors influence many of the topics discussed next. In a changing world that is full of new challenges, the norms and rules of behavior are less clearly determined and more personally defined. While patterns still exist, they're often unique to individuals. A therapist must act flexibly and intelligently with couples, yet he or she is limited by gender, cultural, and social experiences. Selected for discussion are common couple therapy issues that often elicit strong responses from beginning therapists.

Dealing with Infidelity

Disclosure of an affair is a frequent catalyst for couple therapy (Blow & Hartnett, 2005). However, studies attempting to determine the prevalence of affairs have found varied or unclear results ranging from 15 to 65% in heterosexual couples (Blow & Hartnett, 2005; Lawson, 1989). Research indicates that women and men participate in and understand extramarital affairs differently; women tend to engage in emotional relationships while men engage in sexual ones, although this distinction is changing (Brown, 1991; Treas & Giesen, 2000). Also, cross-cultural understanding of infidelity may help a therapist treat the couple more effectively (Penn, Hernandez, & Bermudez, 1997). Finally, treating infidelity with evidence-based practice models is only beginning to be defined (Dupree, White, Olsen, & Lafleur, 2007).

A newer form of infidelity is termed "cyberbetrayal." This type of infidelity is based upon online activity that threatens the couple's relationship. The behaviors can include online infidelity, emotional involvement with potential partners, use of online pornography, involvement in chat rooms, and secretly seeking out potential sexual partners. Cooper (1998) identifies the "triple engine" of access, affordability, and anonymity as primary factors in causing an increase in online cyberbetrayal. The key element in treating this problem is addressing the betrayal. Once it is discovered, most clients feel that their trust has been breached and it must be reestablished. The experience of violation is highly subjective. The person who has been involved in the behavior may minimize the problem, while the other partner usually feels threatened by behavior that they cannot control and often don't understand. The minimization increases their anxiety and creates a polarization (Henline & Howard, 2008).

Two components seem evident in all forms of infidelity: (1) breaking the couple's agreement regarding sexual and/or emotional exclusivity, and (2) secrecy. A partner might react to an "emotional" affair as strongly as to a "physical" affair. The therapist must understand the couple's relational contract and the meaning of the breach of the contract. Therapy could be hindered by not knowing about an affair. Thus, some therapists will ask privately if an individual is engaged in an affair. The risk, however, is that the therapist will be triangulated by one of the partners into keeping the secret from the other. Many marital therapists don't believe that keeping secrets for very long is clinically or ethically responsible behavior. Some choose always to see the couple together and to disclose all information, including telephone conversations, to both partners. Clinicians should be guided by their theoretical orientation and professional or ethical judgment.

If infidelity is identified or disclosed, a crisis intervention often needs to follow. Safety issues, such as suicide risk, should be assessed and dealt with if necessary. Some couples consider separating after the disclosure of the affair. Thus, therapy may need to review some of the pragmatics of life, such as addressing where each partner will be living or sleeping over the next several days, practical care of children and short-term finances. A therapeutic separation (discussed later in this chapter) may be a reasonable response. After this, a clearer definition of the problem can be made to determine if individual or couple therapy should be started. It may be inappropriate to work on the couple's relationship if the affair is continuing. Individual work with a partner who is ambivalent about both marital and extramarital relationships may be necessary before a commitment to couple work is made.

Ending the affair is only the first step in this delicate restoration process. The couple is faced with a number of other tasks: They must find ways to reestablish trust in the relationship; examine the reasons for the affair, which may include both individual and relational factors; provide time for grief and jealousy to be a part of the relationship for a while; and find a way to learn from and let go of (forgive) the infidelity in order to commit to a newly defined relationship (Gordon, Baucom, & Snyder, 2004). When addictive components to the infidelity process are identified, sometimes referral to group or twelve-step programs can assist in the recovery process. In addition, children may have knowledge of the affair or be asked to keep it a secret for a parent, especially if the infidelity has gone on for some time. This might need to be explored.

Domestic Violence

Both in theory and practice, marital and family therapy has only recently begun to fully address domestic violence. It is important that therapists assess all couples for domestic violence. Despite the frequency, potential lethality, and cost of domestic violence, many therapists fail to detect it. In addition, there is continued debate on the best way to treat domestic violence.

As discussed in Chapter 4, the therapist must determine what type of violence is occurring in the relationship since it has important implications for treatment (Greene & Bogo, 2002). It may be possible to conduct couple therapy if the violence falls under the category of common couple violence (sometimes also referred to as situation couple violence). If couple therapy is pursued, it is important that there be a commitment to stopping the violence. If both partners engage in any physical aggression, then both must commit to stopping these actions.

The therapist must also encourage individuals to take full responsibility for their behavior and recognize that violence cannot be part of a healthy relationship. Of course, taking this posture makes it more difficult to therapeutically align with a partner who uses physical aggression. One approach is to discuss with the violent partner how stopping the violence is in his (or her) best interest. The therapist might identify, for example, how continuing the violence damages the individual's relationship with his or her partner, or puts the individual at risk for police involvement.

If you determine that it is safe to do conjoint treatment, then the initial focus is on reducing the risk for violence and ensuring safety. Encouraging couples to take time-outs when emotions rise is an important intervention. Teaching individuals how to self-soothe may be necessary. A referral for anger management is sometimes helpful to supplement the work being done in couple therapy. It is also prudent to have a safety plan in place in the event violence reoccurs. Throughout treatment, you should continually reassess if the couple has experienced any episodes of violence. A subsequent incident of violence during treatment should lead you to reevaluate whether conjoint treatment is contraindicated for the couple.

If the violence falls under the category of patriarchal terrorism (sometimes referred to as intimate terrorism or battering), most clinicians believe couple or conjoint work is contraindicated. The goal at this point is to encourage individuals to seek the appropriate treatment prior to doing couple work. For the violent partner, this may include doing either individual therapy or group therapy for batterers. Victims of domestic violence should be encouraged to develop a safety plan and seek out additional support or resources. Referrals for shelters or legal aid may be necessary.

Therapists need to examine their own beliefs and reactions to domestic violence, especially given its emotional intensity, the potential danger involved, and the effect of any prior victimization of the therapist. Moral, legal, and ethical concerns related to this issue must be well thought out by therapists in order for them to respond professionally. For example, the therapist may have a legal and ethical obligation to file a child abuse report if children witness domestic violence and it leads to emotional or physical harm. Solid supervision must be available when a beginning therapist first encounters this difficult and, sadly, all-too-common aspect of couple work.

Sexual Difficulties

In our role as supervisors, we've found that it's common for beginning therapists to ignore the sexual relationship of their clients. The new therapist often assumes that because the couple doesn't mention problems with sex their sexual relationship is fine. Making such an assumption is a mistake. Many couples that seek therapy are coping with sexual problems and may be waiting for you to ask about the issue because they're too embarrassed or uncomfortable to introduce the concern. A good question to ask when you start your assessment of a couple's sexual relationship is "How does (presenting problem) affect your sexual relationship?" The more comfortable you appear during this assessment, the more likely it is they will reveal the details of their problems (Weeks et al., 2005).

When sexual problems become a focus of your assessment, a sexual history should be taken. Ideally, it's best to explore this history with the couple together and separately. The onset and context of a sexual complaint should be explored so that contributing factors can be clarified. For example, if a man states that he has little desire for sex with his partner, it's important to know if it's a primary problem (no history of sexual desire) or a secondary problem (positive history of sexual desire). In addition, does your client experience feelings of desire in some situations (e.g., during masturbation), or is desire completely absent? Of course, the therapist needs to know if the partners have undergone medical examinations to rule out or clarify any biological causes. It's also important to check if clients are using alcohol, drugs, or prescribed medications that might interfere with sexual functioning. The construction of a sexual genogram (Hof & Berman, 1986) can also be helpful during assessment and treatment to understand sexual beliefs, behaviors, and patterns from each partner's family of origin.

Once you've completed your assessment of a couple's relationship, you'll have some indication of the severity of their sexual issues. For most couples, their sexual problems will comingle with other relationship problems, such as commitment, communication, and conflict management. For other couples, their sexual difficulties will require more significant attention and treatment. Because sex therapy is an advanced skill, you will need to decide if it fits in your scope of competence. If it doesn't, you can refer the couple to a therapist certified by the American Association of Sexuality Educators, Counselors and Therapists (AASECT). At the very least, it's important for you to have a basic understanding of sexual anatomy and physiology, which can usually be acquired in an introductory human sexuality course or in most family therapy training programs.

Gay and Lesbian Couples

Most of the information in this chapter applies to any couple. However, there are some important differences when working with gay and lesbian couples. Table 8.1 provides Green and Mitchell's (2008) summary of common challenges for same-sex couples and suggested interventions. We want to highlight three issues. First, you need to consider the stress encountered by gay and lesbian couples due to prejudice, discrimination, and marginalization in our culture. More than half of the states in the United States carry laws that criminalize forms of sexual expression most common to lesbians and gay men. Data from national lesbian and gay rights organizations shows many gays and lesbians have experienced violence related to their sexual orientation (Franklin & Herek, 2003). Gay and lesbian couples usually cannot designate their partners for work-related benefits or health insurance, nor can they be easily recognized as a legal family member that can visit intensive-care patients or make medical decisions.

A second consideration is the lack of clarity that sometimes exists in gay and lesbian relationships. Unlike heterosexual couples, which have many socially and legally endorsed ways to articulate their commitment to one another (e.g., legal marriage), gay and lesbian couples are not afforded the same kinds of rituals to define their commitment. For example, families of origin frequently shun, distance, ignore, or attack couples attempting to identify and honestly express their commitment, which can leave same-sex couples isolated from broader family ties. Another challenge in defining couple identity is the dearth of relationship role models. Since almost all gays and lesbians grew up in homes dominated by heterosexual relationships, they have few models to draw from in defining roles and responsibilities in their relationships. You can play a helpful role in assisting gay and lesbian couples to clarify their identity as a couple.

A third consideration is the therapist's personal comfort with love, intimacy, and sexuality in gay and lesbian relationships, which Green and Mitchell (2008) consider the most important prerequisite for helping same-sex couples. Personal comfort means appreciation for gay and lesbian culture, the ability to listen empathically to the experiences of gay and lesbian couples, and the willingness to talk about the range of issues that these couples bring to therapy, including sexual difficulties. Therapy with same-sex couples is similar to working cross-culturally with any client: it requires respect for differences and openness to new learning.

The following case example demonstrates that therapy with a lesbian couple, like other family therapy, requires attention to individual, interactional, intergenerational, and community systems.

Susan and Brenda, both in their 40s, have been living together for the past 4 years and were married 3 years ago in a private commitment ceremony. Presenting problems include constant arguing, fre-

TABLE 8.1. Same-Sex Couples in Therapy: Challenges, Problems, Interventions, Goals

Challenges/risk factors	Potential couple problems	Therapeutic interventions	Outcome goals
I. Antigay prejudice in the community and larger society creates minority stress	a. Internalized homophobia—fear and ambivalence about committing to a same-sex couple relationship b. Partner conflicts over how out the couple will be with family, at work, and in the community	a. Externalizing the homophobia—viewing societal ignorance and prejudice (not homosexuality) as a problem b. Negotiating any outness conflicts between partners based on realistic constraints/dangers	a. Self-acceptance of lesbian/gay identity; comfort in committing to a same-sex couple relationship b. Maximizing involvement in social contexts where the couple can be out
II. Lack of normative and legal template for same-sex couplehood	Relational ambiguity (unclear couple commitment, boundaries, expectations, and obligations); insecure attachment in current relationship	Exploration and collaboration about what being a couple means to them (roles, boundaries, mutual obligations); exploring creating legal documents, legalized relationships	Commitment clarity, operating as a team, primary commitment to each other, longer-term planning ability, secure attachment in current relationship
III. Same-sex composition of couple (problematic only if partners are gender conforming)	a. Problems of emotional fusion and avoidance of conflict in female couples b. Problems of emotional disengagement or competition in male couples	Reviewing partners' traditional male or female gender socialization in families of origin and current social contexts; encouraging resistance to and subversion of conventional gender role expectations in the relationship	Androgynous, gender-flexible, egalitarian sharing of emotional and instrumental tasks in the relationship. Collaborative rather than avoidant or competitive approaches to conflict resolution
IV. Lack of social support for the couple relationship	Social isolation; lack of couple identity in a defined community; inability to get emotional support, advice, and instrumental help from a support system	Coaching to build "families of choice" (cohesive social support networks with interconnections among network members)	Embedded couple identity and community of care (social network cohesion, reciprocity of support, higher levels of emotional and instrumental support)

Note. From Green and Mitchell (2008, p. 678). Copyright 2008 by The Guilford Press. Reprinted by permission.

quent conflict, and a lack of intimacy. They say they fight about virtually everything from household responsibilities to money, sex, and how to spend their leisure time. Both report being very dissatisfied with the relationship. The arguments have led to several separations, during which Brenda stayed with her mother. Although neither reports any physical abuse, there have been threats of physical harm, and Brenda reports being afraid of Susan.

The arguments can generate a great deal of emotion, including anger, fear, and rage. Susan says that Brenda is not committed enough to the relationship, that she won't engage enough in discussions about the relationship, and that she withdraws from contact and closeness. Brenda feels intimidated, bullied, criticized, and threatened by Susan. She sees Susan as being unhappy with whatever she does, and feels that she's not ever good enough to meet Susan's high expectations. They do report periods in which they get along well and enjoy each other's company, as long as they keep things superficial.

Susan works full time as an elementary school principal. The job is demanding and she likes it very much. She says that she "gives to others all day long" and wants to be given to at home sometimes. She comes from a family of three children, and is not particularly close to her younger brother and sister. She describes her mother as "good, caring, and warm." Her father physically and verbally abused her. She says that she "still hates him" and is frightened that when she gets angry she becomes just like him. Susan was married to a man when she was 25; the marriage lasted 5 years. She left that relationship for another woman. That partnership lasted 4 years, and was filled with turmoil.

Brenda works part time as a reference librarian. She is an only child and spends much of her time with her ailing grandmother. She has a history of depression and is being treated with antidepressants. During the couple therapy, her depressive symptoms worsened and she felt so overwhelmed that she wasn't able to function in the relationship. She was referred to individual therapy, which proved quite helpful. Brenda feels insecure in the relationship with Susan. She was involved with another woman at the time she met Susan. She reports having felt pressure from Susan to marry.

Susan and Brenda feel frustrated with each other. There has been a lot of blaming and protection of their own feelings. They say they are both committed to the relationship but can't handle the conflict. Their families are supportive and accepting of the relationship. Susan is active in the gay and lesbian community and has been out since her marriage ended. Brenda is out with some friends and family but keeps her sexual orientation a secret at work, which frustrates Susan.

The couple will benefit from discussing their perspectives on being out. It also will be helpful to look at how out they are to their respective families, friends, and work colleagues. The therapist should remain sensitive to their differences and help to mitigate them. Treatment of this couple will need to focus on managing conflict more effectively. Personal and family histories will prove valuable in evaluating their style of conflict and developing some ways to contain and manage it.

Structured Separations

Structured separations may be used either as a possible couple therapy intervention or for couples that are moving toward ending their relationship. A structured separation can be used as a cooling-off period when a couple is involved in intense conflict that isn't currently resolvable. Orderly separations are likely to be less destructive than separations that are disorderly and not anticipated (Ahrons, 1994). Some partners will view any separation as "the end of the marriage" and will have great difficulty with the notion that some structured time apart may be useful. Establishing clear boundaries and negotiating times for contact will be helpful in lowering their anxiety. Expectations regarding visits, telephone contacts, dating, parenting, financial and household responsibilities, and therapy need to be discussed. Specificity in establishing frequency of contacts and who shall initiate the contacts might be necessary.

Therapists need to process both the impact of the couple staying together in an unsatisfying relationship and the family consequences of separation or divorce (Charny, 2006). Nichols (1988) identifies three tasks for the couple involved in the decision to divorce and these same tasks seem appropriate when working with a structured separation:

1. Accepting the reality that a separation/divorce is occurring (regardless of how or by whom the decision is made).
2. Coping with the initial emotional/psychological reactions.
3. Performing the initial planning for the contemplated actions.

The therapist can assist the couple in orchestrating the separation and accomplishing the tasks identified by Nichols.

It is typical for one partner to be asking for a separation while the other desires to stay together and "work things out." A prelude to a prolonged physical separation can be one of the spouses taking a vacation or even structuring time apart. However, if one of the spouses is adamant about insisting upon a separation, then the therapist can be a helpful mediator. The therapist must be sensitive to each person's concerns and avoid developing a coalition with one of the partners.

Evaluating the style and severity of conflict is necessary when working with couples who are separating. If the conflict is severe and chaotic, then the couple should have limited contact and possibly be instructed not to try to solve problems outside therapy, at least initially. If they're less conflicted and able to spend time together in a congenial atmosphere without quickly escalating into difficulties, then they might gradually increase the amount of time they spend together. Spouses need to be able to adhere to the rules of the separation agreement and reestablish trust in each other. If boundaries are violated, then that trust becomes difficult to create. Consequently, rules and boundaries should be fair and realistic for both parties.

WHEN COUPLE THERAPY MIGHT NOT WORK

Couple therapy is not always the therapy of choice. Although therapists might differ in how they decide for or against couple work, several indicators point to the limits of conjoint sessions. One might be the individual pathology presented by one of the partners. For example, severe depression, psychotic thought processes, or active alcoholism or drug abuse in one partner or explosive violence between the couple are potential warning signs that couple therapy might be inappropriate. One way to assess whether presenting problems are conducive to conjoint sessions is to determine if a connection or therapeutic relationship can be made between the therapist and the individual or system. If the therapist fails to develop some structure around the couple's interactions, if one of the pair comes drunk or high to the session, or if an individual's affect so influences the session that it severely hinders any interventions, then the therapist would be wise to separate the couple. A referral of one or both of the partners to other resources before embarking on conjoint therapy may also be considered.

There is wisdom in using individual therapy, or individual group sessions, along with couple therapy. Simultaneously working at an individual and systemic level is merited in complicated cases. The major limits, of course, are the financial and therapeutic resources available for the work to be done. Prioritizing and delineating an overall treatment plan that shows therapy can be provided from different and complementary system levels (biological, individual, relational, cultural) often helps the couple engage in the tough work of therapy. It is important that you review assessment information and treatment planning ideas (Chapter 5) when feeling stuck with a couple.

CONCLUSION

Couple therapy can present several challenges for the beginning therapist. Maintaining a balanced relationship with both partners, building a commitment to therapy if the couple has divergent goals about the relationship, identifying the couple's cycle, and managing the couple's affect are some of the tasks required to do effective therapy with couples. Domestic violence and infidelity can also present challenges in doing couple therapy, and in some cases, may be a contraindication for couple work. However, couple therapy also offers rewards. Given the importance that most people place on having a loving and satisfying intimate relationship with another human being, helping couples achieve this is especially rewarding.

CHAPTER 9

When a Family Member Has a Mental Illness

"I'm convinced there is nothing we cannot cure." One of the authors heard this comment from a senior therapist who had just returned from an upbeat training seminar in the late 1970s. At that time, the author was an inexperienced student therapist. Nevertheless, she questioned the possibility of "cure" for the serious and long-standing struggles her clients faced.

Thirty years later, we have learned that some mental illnesses are intractable despite our best treatment efforts. Families with a mentally ill member may appear at your office door after years of struggle. The illness may have consumed the family's resources and the individual's identity. Nevertheless, family therapists have much to offer these over-extended families. Regardless of the diagnosis, a number of common factors influence families with mentally ill members. Loneliness, lack of social support, and increased stressful life events can make the patient or family's situation worse. Family discord, including frequent hostility, conflict, and overinvolvement can also hurt clients. In contrast, a strong sense of family identity, closeness, and shared values and beliefs can strengthen and protect families. While keeping these relational qualities in mind, family therapists must also know about individual assessment and diagnosis when working with families of the mentally ill.

INDIVIDUAL AND FAMILY CONCEPTS

In the last 20 years, significant gains have been made in describing mental disorders and discovering effective treatments. The National Institute of Mental Health (NIMH) has sponsored important research examining mental disorders that affect millions of people. Some of this work has looked at promising new treatments such as cognitive-behavioral therapy for anxiety disorders or psychoeducational approaches for bipolar disorder (Miklowitz, 2008). New research initiatives are being encouraged in the realm of child and adolescent disorders (Rapee, Wignall, Spence, Cobham, & Lyneham, 2008).

A growing body of literature examines research on effective treatments for individual disorders. Cognitive-behavioral treatments, interpersonal treatments, and family-based treatments have been used in field trials for specific disorders. There is a growing awareness that one treatment might not work for every problem, and a current trend to match specific therapies with certain disorders. In addition, there is a growing focus on prevention, especially for children and adolescents. As we learn more about gene–environment interactions, clinicians hope that early interventions, at the onset of mental health problems, can protect the child and keep the illness from worsening.

In addition to the research on talk therapies, there is a burgeoning literature on the effectiveness of pharmacological treatments. New medications are coming out almost daily to treat disorders that were once considered untreatable. The introduction of Prozac created a public awareness of psychopharmacological medications, and people began to demand the pills that reputedly could change a personality and transform a life. Current research is looking at the efficacy of a "split treatment model"—a combination of talk therapy and medication. Other research examines how an individual's genetics may influence his or her response to psychotropic medication.

We now know that mental illness can run in families and that transmission may not only result from dysfunctional family patterns, but also involve biological determinants. More often than not, when one mentions family history in a psychological assessment, it refers to genetic transmission. Individual diagnosticians are very interested in relatives both in the present and past who have a history of mental illness because this suggests genetic transmission in the patient.

Research on genetic transmission was enlightening news to families of the mentally ill. After years of subtly being blamed for their family members' problems through concepts such as the "schizophrenogenic mother," families were both saddened and relieved to learn the illness has a genetic component. While these discoveries relieve the family of guilt and responsibility for "causing" mental illnesses, they also can transmit some discouraging news about prognosis and transmission to future generations.

Families will be interested to know that while they did not cause mental illness in one member, they can influence its course. Research on "expressed emotion" and "communication deviance" in schizophrenic families demonstrates that family qualities like overinvolvement, hostility, and critical attitudes can influence the schizophrenic family member to relapse. More recently, emotional dysregulation, hostility, and conflict in the family have been examined in relation to depression, dementia, schizophrenia, and a variety of other disorders (Miklowitz, 2008; Beach & Jones, 2002; Gross, 2007). This research has demonstrated the powerful impact family behaviors and mood can have on individual members and their illnesses.

Family therapists can consider psychiatric consultation for the family member with mental illness. The consultation can provide information that the therapist can integrate into the overall treatment plan. In addition, the psychiatrist might recommend psychotropic medication to treat the symptoms of the individual's mental disorder.

Beginning family therapists can glean useful therapeutic tools from the world of individual diagnosis and simultaneously incorporate the strengths of family therapy. Therapists do not need to choose one ideological position to the exclusion of all other perspectives. Beginning family therapists can use multiple sources of information and perspectives to create an optimal treatment plan for their clients.

Even if you recognize the key concepts of individual diagnosis or family process, it can still be overwhelming to sort out the distinctions when you are doing assessment. A suicidal teenager who is not sleeping or eating because she is upset about her grades and her parents' fighting may be hard to identify when her parents bring her to see you "because she is just not motivated in school." In fact, a common struggle that new therapists face is sorting through the family's view of the problems, the referral source's views, and individual members' views. Discernment about assessment and treatment can be especially challenging if you are unfamiliar with individual diagnostic criteria or if you hold personal allegiance to one school of therapy.

One of the most common struggles we observe in new students is their ready acceptance of the problem definition, especially if an authority such as a parent, school principal, or physician refers the family for a specific, detailed problem. In addition, if a couple or family come for therapy and define the problem relationally, the therapist may be reluctant to consider individual diagnoses. In like manner, if the family describes the problem as a problem with an individual, the therapist may be averse to exploring family dynamics. We observed a diagnostic challenge when a couple came for marital therapy because they were fighting. The wife's complaints included the husband's disorganization, inability to be on time, inability to keep a job, and explosive anger. While the therapist started working on conflict resolution and communication skills with the couple, he also noted the husband's chaotic life. The husband was never on time to the sessions and on several occasions forgot the session entirely, even when the wife reminded him the day before. After a while, the therapist began to wonder if the husband had attention deficit disorder. While maintaining a focus on the couple, the therapist gently explored the husband's learning history more carefully. Ultimately, a diagnosis of adult ADHD resulted in dramatic changes in the husband's life, the wife's life, and the marriage.

INDIVIDUAL DIAGNOSIS IN A FAMILY CONTEXT

Epidemiological research suggests that more than 50% of the population will have a mental disorder at some time in their lives (Kessler et al., 2005). While this statistic may refer to a problem as simple as an adjustment disorder, the frequency of mental health problems suggests the need for effective treatments. While most people who have a mental health problem improve spontaneously and without treatment, there is a small minority, approximately 14%, who have recurring episodes of mental illness, often at least three major episodes during their lifetime. Researchers and clinicians also note that one patient frequently has several problems (comorbidity). Epidemiological data and clinical experience suggest that mental problems of various durations and intensities are frequent, debilitating, and painful for both the person and his or her family (Kessler et al., 1994, 2005).

People often have mental health problems that do not meet DSM-IV-TR diagnostic criteria. The individual diagnostician who closely follows DSM-IV-TR diagnostic outlines risks overlooking serious problems that do not fit neatly into a category. This poses a more serious risk for children and adolescents because their problems fit DSM-IV-TR criteria less frequently than adult disorders and can be strongly influenced by developmental issues that might be overlooked by the diagnostician completing a DSM symptom checklist. A contextual, holistic approach to mental health problems can correct for many of these weaknesses.

The most common DSM-IV-TR disorders are mood disorders (such as depression), anxiety disorders, and substance abuse problems. Frequently, a patient suffers from two or more of these disorders simultaneously. While everyone suffers from depression or anxiety at some time in his or her life, illness does not refer to these everyday problems but to known, recognizable syndromes. Specificity of symptoms, duration, and intensity distinguish a syndrome from the common problems of living.

However, clinicians and patients often find the distinction between a syndrome and everyday problems unilluminating. A patient who is going through a divorce, working as a single parent, and worried about losing her job doesn't care whether she meets four or five criteria for major depression to justify this diagnosis. She just wants to feel better. In addition, patients with non-DSM-IV-TR problems such as chronic pain, marital problems, or physical illness simply want relief, not a diagnosis.

As a result, clinicians primarily use DSM-IV-TR when it comes to filling out forms or for reimbursement purposes. However, when doing treatment, they focus on the most comprehensive view of the problem(s), which often expands beyond a DSM-IV-TR diagnosis. While the vast majority of family therapists are trained in individual diagnosis (Denton et al., 1997), they may initially disregard individual symptom assessment in order to obtain a more holistic understanding of the patient and his or her family's problems, and to briefly enter the patient's world with as few distractions as possible (Beach & Gupta, 2005).

The practical, ethical, and logistical dilemmas of using both individual and family diagnosis have never been clearly delineated. Family therapists have discussed some of the inherent strengths and weaknesses of combining individual and family approaches in assessment and treatment (Beach & Jones, 2002; Beach et al., 2006). For the most part, the family therapist has been left the task of working out the nuances of integrating these approaches. How can a family therapist effectively integrate information on individual diagnosis and still maintain a systemic, contextual, holistic perspective? Perhaps this can be done by maintaining an attitude of openness—a willingness to consider the possibility of individual diagnosis while still maintaining the strengths of a family therapy approach.

Research on health and illness suggests that loneliness, together with lack of social support, is one of the strongest predictors of decline and further suffering, regardless of the problem. Loss of an important relationship through death, divorce, or other means is rated as one of the most significant stressors a person can experience. Family therapy's strength is its recognition of the importance of these relationships, regardless of the other mental health problems an individual experiences. Being isolated and having no social support can signal problems.

Research on bipolar illness and other affective disorders suggests that while individual symptoms can be recognized and perhaps treated with medication or by other means, the symptomatic person still desires the support and love of family (Clarkin & Glick, 1992; Beach & Gupta, 2006; Miklowitz, 2008). In addition, the individual can be either hurt or helped by familial responses. A family therapist can successfully combine, in his or her work, the basic tenets of systemic thinking with careful attention to individual problems and the clinical literature on both systemic and individual perspectives.

Clearly, the therapist must pay attention to the symptoms of the identified patient as well as to the characteristics and symptoms of other family members. Questions to think about include the following: "Does this person have a known, recognizable cluster of symptoms that meet specific diagnostic criteria?" "Should this individual receive treatment for these symptoms, in addition to any other therapeutic goals?" "Do I, as the therapist, have the skills and knowledge to recognize and treat this problem, or should I consider referral to someone else?"

While most family therapists can recognize symptoms of common problems such as depression or anxiety, they may not spot less frequently occurring syndromes. For example, family therapy students may be unfamiliar with signs indicating Tourette's syndrome or trichotillomania. There are several remedies for this situation.

First, family therapists should make every effort to keep up with the literature on individual diagnoses. In addition, they can maintain an attitude of curiosity and alertness to clinical situations they haven't encountered in the past. Frequent reflection on one's clinical caseload and increased supervision for beginning therapists invite further exploration of clinically unfamiliar situations. When the unusual happens, the therapist can begin by consulting colleagues and reading.

Referral to a psychotherapist with expertise in a specific diagnosis is always an option. For example, many family therapists will not treat a family whose adolescent has an eating disorder unless they have significant previous experience in that area. They recognize the severity of the condition, and while they may continue family therapy for other issues or related problems, they make sure the adolescent gets an appropriate referral to a psychotherapist or physician who knows how to treat eating disorders.

Finally, family therapists need to be aware of individual diagnoses because the healthcare system demands it. As more therapists are paid by the government or other large payer organizations, they will be expected to diagnose and plan treatment according to commonly accepted protocol. Even when family therapy is a common and highly regarded treatment, familiarity with individual diagnoses will be essential to obtain treatment authorization and fulfill insurance form requirements.

While it would be impossible to describe every individual problem and its treatment here, the rest of this chapter focuses on four of
the most common individual disorders: depression, anxiety, substance
abuse, and impulse control. These disorders are the most commonly
occurring ones in the general population, and often disorders start at
a young age (See Table 9.1). At times, these problems are described as
discrete entities, but family therapists recognize that even these disorders are best viewed in a holistic context. A contextual approach makes
room for consideration of primary symptoms, other social and emotional problems, and the family's extant strengths and deficits.

TABLE 9.1. Most Common Mental Health Disorders

Disorder	Prevalence	Mean age at onset
Anxiety	28%	11 years
Impulse (ODD, CD, ADHD)	25%	11 years
Mood	21%	30 years
Substance	15%	20 years
All disorders	46%	½ by 14 years; ¾ by 24 years

Do patients seeks help and when?

Disorder	What percentage ever seek help	Wait how long after onset of symptoms
Anxiety	60	9–23 years
Mood	88	6–8 years
Impulse	40	
Substance	40	

Predictors of *not* seeking treatment: early age of onset, elderly, male, married, low education, minority.

Who receives the most treatment? Patients with comorbid illnesses—7% of population with three or more diagnoses.

Predictors of never getting treatment: elderly, minorities, poor, no insurance, rural patients.

Note. Data from Kessler, Berglund, et al. (2005) and Kessler, Chiu, Demler, and Walters (2005).

Two other disorders that we do not describe in much detail but deserve mentioning are psychotic disorders and somatization disorders. While being able to treat patients with psychotic disorders is a critical skill, these treatments are not covered in detail in this book because psychoses are less common than other disorders. Nevertheless, we recommend that all family therapists recognize the hallmark signs and symptoms of psychoses: hallucinations, delusions, loss of interest in life, changing speech patterns, and a flat mood. Hallucinations refer to sensory experiences and the most common hallucination is hearing voices. Delusions refer to false beliefs, for instance, believing that your neighbor has implanted a radio in your head. If you are treating any family members that complain of these symptoms or have other types of odd thinking, it is time to refer the patient to a psychiatrist for a more careful evaluation. (Suggestions for working with physicians and more information about psychoses and other major mental illnesses are described in *The Therapist's Guide to Psychopharmacology* by Patterson, Albala, MacCahill, & Edwards, 2006.)

Referral to a psychiatrist does not mean that you will no longer treat the patient and his or her family. Often, once a psychotic patient's most disruptive symptoms are treated, usually by medication, the family is at a loss for how to proceed. Diagnosis of a major mental illness such as psychosis can be a devastating experience for a family. They may wonder what to expect in the future, feel impatient, and even angry with the patient. Family therapists can play a significant role in helping families deal with the day-to-day challenges of coping with mental illness. Families need information about what to expect and they need another asset that you can provide—hope. If you become knowledgeable about psychoses, you can guide the family through many challenges. Often, the challenges deal with boundaries, both real and interpersonal. For example, clients wonder where their ill family member should live, or they may experience interpersonal problems such as feeling irritated or embarrassed by the ill member's strange behaviors. It is not uncommon for families to feel abandoned by the mental health system once the patient has received a diagnosis and medication. Before clients begin feeling abandoned, you can offer education, guidance, hope, structure, and the support of a therapeutic relationship that might last for many years.

The second diagnosis that we do not describe in detail is somatization disorder. Instead of referring to the specific disorder, we want to focus on somatizing symptoms, regardless of the diagnosis. "Somatic" means "relating to or affecting the body." As part of a holistic, biopsychosocial approach, therapists are interested in patients' physical symptoms, not just their relationships or thoughts. While you want to remain aware of scope-of-practice issues and not treat a problem outside your expertise, many physical symptoms are one part of a carousel of issues you can address. Depending on the circumstances, physical symptoms may demand immediate attention. For example, a depressed patient may not be able to sleep. An anxious patient may be losing weight because he has lost his appetite. A wife may no longer be interested in sexual relations regardless of her husband's efforts.

Regardless of the individual or family diagnosis, prominent physical symptoms deserve the therapist's attention, even if only for a referral to a physician. Physical symptoms may indicate a much larger problem, such as clinical depression or substance abuse. In addition, physical symptoms including sexual problems, chronic pain, eating problems, and sleep problems may become, at least temporarily, the focus of treatment. It is not necessary for you to be an expert in all areas. Instead, you simply need the skills to recognize these issues when they arise in the session, make them a clinical focus, and know how to enlist help from colleagues like physicians when the problems are outside your expertise. In addition, you can encourage your patients to take a holistic approach to their health. While you continue to focus on family dynamics and individual psychopathology, you can encourage your patients to exercise, lose weight, or smoke less—general health habits that are known to affect both physical and mental health.

DEPRESSION

When individual diagnosticians talk about mood disorders, they refer to specific criteria or symptoms—something beyond the "blues" that everyone experiences at one time or another. The most common syndromes include bipolar disorder, cyclothymia, dysthymia, and major depression (Belmaker & Agam, 2008). Depressive symptoms appear in other disorders, such as atypical depression, adjustment disorder with depressed mood, and schizoaffective disorder, but describing these varied conditions is beyond the scope of this book. For family therapists, it is important to note that child and adolescent depression have different pathways and presentations. For example, depression in children frequently presents with irritability.

The prevalence of depression in the general population is high and on the rise (Belmaker & Agam, 2008; Kessler et al., 2005). Up to one in eight individuals may require treatment for depression in their lifetime. However, the majority of depressed people never receive any treatment; if they do, it is usually from their primary care physician, not a family therapist.

Besides being painful, depression can be debilitating and recurring. Bipolar depression is characterized by swings between elated moods (manic or hypomanic episodes) and depressed moods, while cyclothymia is characterized by a more mild manifestation of the same swings. Dysthymia refers to a type of depression that has lasted for at least 2 years and whose symptoms are less debilitating than major depression. Major depression, meanwhile, is a condition in which intense feelings of sadness, loss, and helplessness prevail, to the point of impairing daily functioning. Table 9.2 provides a quick reference for mood disorders, as well as diagnostic criteria for major depressive episodes and manic episodes.

Depression occurs twice as often in women as in men (McGrath, Keita, Strickland, & Russon, 1990; Denton & Burwell, 2006). Possible explanations include women's characteristic style of internalizing problems (thinking instead of doing) compared to men's more aggressive and externalizing style. The social circumstances of women (living in poverty, or suffering abuse) also play a role. Many mental health experts consider depression in women almost epidemic.

Major risk factors for depression include a family history of depression (regardless of whether this is due to interactional or biological factors), lack of social support, stressful life events, and suicides by family members. In addition, depression frequently is found in individuals who suffer from anxiety or have substance abuse problems. While most patients recover from depression without treatment, they are at high risk for relapse. In addition, the most rigorous study ever completed on treatment for depression found that only 19–32% of recovered patients stayed well for more than a year (Shea, Gibbons, Elkin, & Sotsky, 1995; Patterson et al., 2006).

The symptoms of bipolar illness (manic-depressive disorder) are often dramatic and intense, and the majority of bipolar patients will experience about 11 episodes of either mania (elated mood) or depression (sad, tearful, hopeless mood) during their lifetime (Miklowitz, 2008). In addition, manic-depressive illness is seldom "cured," but managed throughout a person's life. A family who witnesses an initial episode in one of its members can expect more of the same in years to come. These bouts can leave a family reeling and wondering when the next "crazy" episode will happen. One family powerfully described their confusion when police told them that their college-age son threw a microwave oven through a store window. Their story chronicles years of treatment, confusion, feeling blamed, and eventual healing after their son was diagnosed with bipolar illness (Berger & Berger, 1991).

TABLE 9.2. Quick Reference for Mood Disorders

Disorder	Description
Major depressive disorder	Characterized by one or more major depressive episodes (i.e., at least 2 weeks of depressed mood or loss of interest accompanied by at least four additional symptoms of depression).
Dysthymic disorder	Characterized by at least 2 years of depressed mood for more days than not, accompanied by additional depressive symptoms that do not meet criteria for a major depressive episode.
Bipolar I disorder	Characterized by one or more manic or mixed episodes, usually accompanied by major depressive episodes.
Bipolar II disorder	Characterized by one or more major depressive episodes accompanied by at least one hypomanic episode.
Cyclothymic disorder	Characterized by at least 2 years of numerous periods of hypomanic symptoms that do not meet criteria for a manic episode and numerous periods of depressive symptoms that do not meet criteria for a major depressive episode.

Criteria for major depressive episode[a]

A. Five (or more) of the following symptoms have been present during the same 2-week period and represent a change from previous functioning; at least one of the symptoms is either (1) depressed mood or (2) loss of interest or pleasure....

   (1) depressed mood most of the day, nearly every day, as indicated by either subjective report (e.g., feels sad or empty) or observation made by others (e.g., appears tearful). **Note:** In children and adolescents, can be irritable mood.
   (2) markedly diminished interest or pleasure in all, or almost all, activities most of the day, nearly every day (as indicated by either subjective account or observation made by others)
   (3) significant weight loss when not dieting or weight gain (e.g., a change of more than 5% of body weight in a month), or decrease or increase in appetite nearly every day. **Note:** In children, consider failure to make expected weight gains.
   (4) insomnia or hypersomnia nearly every day
   (5) psychomotor agitation or retardation nearly every day (observable by others, not merely subjective feelings of restlessness or being slowed down)
   (6) fatigue or loss of energy nearly every day
   (7) feelings of worthlessness or excessive or inappropriate guilt (which may be delusional) nearly every day (not merely self-reproach or guilt about being sick)
   (8) diminished ability to think or concentrate, or indecisiveness, nearly every day (either by subjective account or as observed by others)
   (9) recurrent thoughts of death (not just fear of dying), recurrent suicidal ideation without a specific plan, or a suicide attempt or specific plan for committing suicide

(cont.)

TABLE 9.2. *(cont.)*

B. The symptoms do not meet criteria for a mixed episode.

C. The symptoms cause clinically significant distress or impairment in social, occupational, or other important areas of functioning.

D. The symptoms are not due to the direct physiological effects of a substance (e.g., a drug of abuse, a medication) or a general medical condition (e.g., hypothyroidism).

E. The symptoms are not better accounted for by bereavement (i.e., after the loss of a loved one). The symptoms persist for longer than 2 months or are characterized by marked functional impairment, morbid preoccupation with worthlessness, suicidal ideation, psychotic symptoms, or psychomotor retardation.

Criteria for manic episode[b]

A. A distinct period of abnormally and persistently elevated, expansive, or irritable mood, lasting at least 1 week (or any duration if hospitalization is necessary).

B. During the period of mood disturbance, three (or more) of the following symptoms have persisted (four if the mood is only irritable) and have been present to a significant degree:

  (1) inflated self-esteem or grandiosity
  (2) decreased need for sleep (e.g., feels rested after only 3 hours of sleep)
  (3) more talkative than usual or pressure to keep talking
  (4) flight of ideas or subjective experience that thoughts are racing
  (5) distractibility (i.e., attention too easily drawn to unimportant or irrelevant external stimuli)
  (6) increase in goal-directed activity (either socially, at work or school, or sexually) or psychomotor agitation
  (7) excessive involvement in pleasurable activities that have a high potential for painful consequences (e.g., engaging in unrestrained buying sprees, sexual indiscretions, or foolish business investments)

C. The symptoms do not meet criteria for a mixed episode.

D. The mood disturbance is sufficiently severe to cause marked impairment in occupational functioning or in usual social activities or relationships with others, or to necessitate hospitalization to prevent harm to self or others, or there are psychotic features.

E. The symptoms are not due to the direct physiological effects of a substance (e.g., a drug of abuse, a medication, or other treatment) or a general medical condition (e.g., hyperthyroidism).

[a]From American Psychiatric Association (2000, p. 356). Copyright 2000 by the American Psychiatric Association. Reprinted by permission.
[b]From American Psychiatric Association (2000, p. 362). Copyright 2000 by the American Psychiatric Association. Reprinted by permission.

Family therapy has been examined as a treatment for major depression and dysthymia, and researchers have explored using couple group therapy in cases where one member of the dyad has bipolar disorder (Clarkin & Glick, 1992; Moltz, 1993; Beach & Jones, 2002; Cordova & Gee, 2001). A close relationship with a depressed person is difficult at best. The relationship can be challenged by the sad, hopeless quality the depressed person emanates or the dramatic swings in mood and behavior of the bipolar patient. In addition, the depressed person may look to significant others to help them cope or, even worse, they may withdraw from relationships completely.

The family's response to the depressed person can be a key influence on the course of the depression (Kung, 2000; MacFarlane, 2003). Some research on depression has examined marital therapy, especially behavioral marital therapy, as a form of treatment (Beach & Jones, 2002; Uebelacker, Weishaar, & Miller, 2008). Results of these outcome studies demonstrate that for adults who received marital therapy to treat depression, the marriage improved and the depression abated. Treating depression with marital therapy makes sense, especially when one considers that the most prevalent patient is a wife or mother, in her late 20s to early 40s, who is socially isolated and depressed about her relationship with her husband.

In discussing social and family relationships of depressed persons, Gotlib and Beach (1995) state:

> Whereas depressed persons exhibit social skills deficits in their interactions with strangers, their interactions with their spouse and children are more likely to be characterized by hostility and anger ... it is clear that depression in one family member has a significant influence on the emotions and behavior of other members and ... on the family as a unit. Conversely, negative interactions with spouse or other family members are powerfully related to level of depressive symptomatology. (p. 418)

While no research suggests that families cause depression in individuals, studies indicate that family members affect the course of the illness (Keitner, Ryan, Miller, & Kohn, 1993; Beach & Gupta, 2006). Many researchers suggest a reciprocal relationship between depression and family interaction, stating that it is impossible to identify a single etiology. However, researchers agree that empathic family support can play a critical role in healing. On the negative side, criticism and continued hostility seem to have a harmful effect on both the depressed person and the family. For women, equality in decision making and companionship in marriage protect against depression and a variety of other health problems (Cohen, 2004). In addition, some research suggests that depressed patients tend to relapse at lower levels of criticism than do schizophrenic patients (Keitner et al., 1993). Clearly, family support (especially spousal support) is critical in the course and treatment of depression (Miklowitz, 2008; Cordova & Gee, 2001).

For some couples, spouses of depressed persons may be empathic to their partner's suffering at first but over time become impatient and even hostile. The therapist and family confront a challenging situation when the hostile spouse identifies the reason for that hostility as the partner's helpless behavior and the depressed spouse claims a need for the partner's love and support to improve. The influence of criticism, contempt, defensiveness, and withdrawal in couples with a depressed partner are important because these same themes predict marital deterioration and divorce (Gottman, 1994). In addition, distress and psychopathology in parents predict the same in children. Depression is not an isolated illness residing within an individual, but a serious condition that affects every family relationship, and even the continuing existence of the family.

Family therapists can empathize with the burden spouses feel in helping the depressed client. Common issues family members may present with include the degree of responsibility one must assume for the depressed member, suppressing or denying one's own feelings or needs, generalizing the illness and blaming all negative behaviors and family interactions on it, and arguing with the spouse about treatment recommendations such as medication compliance and therapy.

A family therapist's ability to provide support, education, and information about depression can affect not only the individual patient but the marital and parenting relationships as well. Family therapists can assess not only for the individual symptoms of depression but for the impact the depressed person's mood and behaviors have on other family members and the group's overall well-being. Spouses and children of depressed parents can be considered an integral part of the treatment.

In particular, the intertwined relationships among an individual's depression (especially a woman's), the marriage, and parenting need careful examination. Treatment should be multifaceted, addressing each of these issues and their overlap. There may be no other mental disorder whose course has been demonstrated to have as clear a relationship to marital quality as depression. In addition, children's therapists lament that adult therapists often overlook the impact of parental problems on children's development. Family therapists treating depressed parents have the opportunity to assess and treat the children who are affected by their parents' emotional states.

Studies looking at a marital format to treat depression suggest that women with unipolar depression, who are distressed about their marriage, can be effectively treated with marital therapy (Prince & Jacobson, 1995; Beach & Gupta, 2006). The patient's perception of the problem is important in deciding what type of treatment to pursue. The therapist can assess how central the marital relationship is in the patient's beliefs about why she is depressed.

Evidence suggests that parent–child disputes are prominent in families with a depressed member (Gotlib & Beach, 1995; Uebelacker et al., 2008), and that depressed children grow up in homes with one or more depressed parents. Thus, family therapy can potentially ameliorate a damaging situation for multiple family members, not only treating the individual symptoms of the depressed person but also potentially improving the marriage and the parent–child relationships.

Current research and information about depression give beginning family therapists several guidelines to follow when working with depressed people and their families:

- Check for a family history of depression.
- Consider medication for the depressed family member as an efficient, cost-effective treatment option.
- Consider how the marital relationship influences the member's depression (by asking him or her).
- Note other family members' responses to the depressed member (e.g., distancing, empathizing, hostility, overinvolvement, criticism).
- When a parent is depressed, assess the impact on the children.
- Look for depression masked as other symptoms (e.g., irritability, anger, withdrawal).
- Consider treatment options including individual therapy (especially cognitive-behavioral treatments), couple therapy, family therapy, and group therapy, and match treatment to the specific needs and wishes of the clients.
- Use psychoeducation to inform family members about depression.

Marital and family therapies to treat depression generally work best for clients with mild depression and have been shown to be less effective for those who were part of an inpatient sample of severely depressed persons (Prince & Jacobson, 1995). Marital and family therapies may be used in conjunction with other treatments, such as pharmacotherapy and/or individual therapy.

ANXIETY

Everyone gets anxious and nervous at times—it's the human condition. But true anxiety disorders are more intense and specific than the general worry we all experience. Fortunately, treatments for these disorders have some of the most successful outcome evidence. New work is going on daily in discovering better pharmacological and cognitive-behavioral treatments for anxiety disorders and much has been learned about emotion regulation and anxiety in recent years (Amstadter, 2008; Gross, 2007). While most mental health problems have a 50–70% treatment success rate, some of the anxiety disorders have a 70–90% cure rate, particularly panic attack with agoraphobia. With these statistics in mind, a family therapist might consider referral to an individual therapist with expertise in pharmacology or cognitive-behavioral treatments for the individual, while simultaneously continuing to treat the family.

Not all anxiety disorders can be treated effectively, however, and recent research suggests that changes in the brain are associated with some anxiety disorders (Etkin & Wager, 2007). For example, posttraumatic stress disorder is often difficult to cure but can be managed. Nevertheless, compared to many disorders where the goal is symptom management, one can, at times, talk about cure for some anxiety disorders. Major subtypes of anxiety disorders, as well as diagnostic criteria for two of these (panic attack and generalized anxiety disorder) are highlighted in Table 9.3.

Frequently, people suffer from both an anxiety disorder and another major problem, such as depression or substance abuse. At times, a client may suffer from all three, using the substance to deal with the other two problems. Physicians who prescribe medication often try to delineate the specific symptoms of each disorder, and prescribe medication to treat them. They also try to understand which cluster of symptoms is dominant. Thus the patient's primary diagnosis might be generalized anxiety disorder with symptoms of depression.

These distinctions, while important, may be less critical to a family therapist. While the therapist can profit from identifying specific symptoms of each disorder, the client is treated as a whole person, and symptoms are seen as part of a whole life, not discrete entities. The patient's perspective and family context are equally important.

Anxiety disorders are common, and occur almost twice as often in women than in men (Castle, Kulkarni, & Abel, 2006). Prevalence of anxiety disorders does not vary, however, on the basis of race, income, education, or rural versus urban living. Once again, we note that women tend to internalize (and become anxious) while men are

TABLE 9.3. Quick Reference for Anxiety Disorders

Disorder	Description
Panic attack	A discrete period in which there is the sudden onset of intense apprehension, fearfulness, or terror, often associated with feelings of impending doom. See criteria for panic attack for specific symptoms.
Agoraphobia	Anxiety about, or avoidance of, places or situations from which escape might be difficult (or embarrassing) or in which help may not be available in the event of a panic attack or panic-like symptoms.
Panic disorder	Without agoraphobia, is characterized by recurrent unexpected panic attacks about which there is persistent concern. With agoraphobia, is characterized by both recurrent, unexpected panic attacks and agoraphobia. Without a history of panic disorder, is characterized by agoraphobia and panic-like symptoms.
Specific phobia	Is characterized by clinically significant anxiety provoked by exposure to a specific feared object or situation, often leading to avoidance behavior.
Social phobia	Is characterized by clinically significant anxiety provoked by exposure to certain types of social or performance situations, often leading to avoidance behavior.
Obsessive-compulsive disorder	Is characterized by obsessions (which cause marked anxiety or distress) and/or by compulsions (which serve to neutralize anxiety).
Posttraumatic stress disorder	Is characterized by the reexperiencing of an extremely traumatic event accompanied by symptoms of increased arousal and by avoidance of stimuli associated with the trauma.
Acute stress disorder	Is characterized by symptoms similar to those of posttraumatic stress disorder that occur immediately in the aftermath of an extremely traumatic event.
Generalized anxiety disorder	Is characterized by at least 6 months of persistent and excessive anxiety and worry.

Criteria for panic attack[a]

A discrete period of intense fear or discomfort, in which four (or more) of the following symptoms developed abruptly and reached a peak within 10 minutes:

    (1) palpitations, pounding heart, or accelerated heart rate
    (2) sweating
    (3) trembling or shaking
    (4) sensations of shortness of breath or smothering
    (5) feeling of choking
    (6) chest pain or discomfort

(cont.)

TABLE 9.3. *(cont.)*

(7) nausea or abdominal distress
(8) feeling dizzy, unsteady, lightheaded, or faint
(9) derealization (feelings of unreality) or depersonalization (being detached from oneself)
(10) fear of losing control or going crazy
(11) fear of dying
(12) paresthesias (numbness or tingling sensations)
(13) chills or hot flushes

Criteria for generalized anxiety disorder[b]

A. Excessive anxiety and worry (apprehensive expectation), occurring more days than not for at least 6 months, about a number of events or activities (such as work or school performance).

B. The person finds it difficult to control the worry.

C. The anxiety and worry are associated with three (or more) of the following six symptoms (with at least some symptoms present for more days than not for the past 6 months). **Note:** Only one item is required in children.

(1) restlessness or feeling keyed up or on edge
(2) being easily fatigued
(3) difficulty concentrating or mind going blank
(4) irritability
(5) muscle tension
(6) sleep disturbance (difficulty falling or staying asleep, or restless, unsatisfying sleep)

D. The focus of the anxiety and worry is not confined to features of an Axis I disorder, that is, the anxiety or worry is not about having a panic attack (as in panic disorder), being embarrassed in public (as in social phobia), being contaminated (as in obsessive-compulsive disorder), being away from home or close relatives (as in separation anxiety disorder), gaining weight (as in anorexia nervosa), having multiple physical complaints (as in somatization disorder), or having a serious illness (as in hypochondriasis), and the anxiety and worry do not occur exclusively during posttraumatic stress disorder.

E. The anxiety, worry, or physical symptoms cause clinically significant distress or impairment in social, occupational, or other important areas of functioning.

F. The disturbance is not due to the direct physiological effects of a substance (e.g., a drug of abuse, a medication) or a general medical condition (e.g., hyperthyroidism) and does not occur exclusively during a mood disorder, a psychotic disorder, or a pervasive developmental disorder.

[a]From American Psychiatric Association (2000, p. 432). Copyright 2000 by the American Psychiatric Association. Reprinted by permission.
[b]From American Psychiatric Association (2000, p. 476). Copyright 2000 by the American Psychiatric Association. Reprinted by permission.

more likely to externalize or act (perhaps get drunk or become violent) when they are distressed.

Anxiety disorders are the most frequently diagnosed problem of children and adolescents, and some research suggests that anxious children become anxious adults (Dadds, 1995; Kessler et al., 2005; Beidel & Turner, 2007). Children's worries are different from adults', and they have different kinds of fears. They may not want to go to school (school phobia), they may be afraid of strangers, or they may not want to leave their mothers (separation anxiety). Regardless of the age-appropriate symptoms, anxiety in childhood can be a frightening and debilitating problem.

Since anxiety disorders generally involve how or what an individual is thinking and his or her physiological responses to these thoughts, it's easy to understand why they might be thought of as problems of the individual. Indeed, sometimes anxiety disorders can be effectively and efficiently treated with individual therapies. Pharmacological treatments and cognitive-behavioral treatments are effective for people suffering from anxiety, and have little or no focus on the patient's family.

Cognitive-behavioral treatments focus on changing how people think and behave. An underlying assumption is that if a person changes thinking or behavior, physiology and emotions will change, too. Gradually exposing someone to the situation they most fear and giving them new ways of thinking about it have proven especially useful treatments.

These methods are similar to the structural family therapy techniques of reframing and enactment. In addition, solution-focused therapists suggest "making one small change" in the way one normally behaves regarding a problem. Narrative therapists talk about someone's "inner dialogue" and "re-storying" one's life. These family therapy approaches share many similarities with cognitive-behavioral techniques.

The major focus for marital therapy in anxiety disorders is often agoraphobia and panic. New research is just beginning to incorporate spouses in the treatment of obsessive-compulsive disorder, social phobia, generalized anxiety disorder, and posttraumatic stress disorder. Existing evidence on outcomes for these disorders suggests that social support—especially family support—leads to superior outcomes. Negative family interactions—such as criticism, anger, hostile confrontation, and a spouse's belief that the client could control his or her own symptoms if he or she wished—were all predictors of poor outcome (Craske & Zoellner, 1995; Gross, 2007; Kase & Ledley, 2007; McLean, Miller, McLean, Chodkiewicz, & Whittal, 2006).

The role of family therapy may be even stronger when treating children with anxiety disorders. Research suggests that fearful, apprehensive responses instead of feelings of mastery and competence are learned by children—often by watching their parents (Morris & March, 2004; Beidel & Turner, 2007). Some research suggests that anxious children grow up in homes with at least one anxious parent. While the family therapist needs to be careful not to fall into the historical trap of blaming the parents for the origins of the child's problems, he or she needs to understand how each parent responds to anxiety-producing stimuli and what the family's response to fearful situations has been in the past. Family treatments, especially those employing cognitive-behavioral principles, can be effective since family members share many beliefs, including a worldview. In addition, the powerful influence of emotional support of spouses and parents can be directed toward recognizing and praising mastery and competence instead of reinforcing worry.

Family therapists are aware of covert and overt rules and beliefs in the family as well as hidden agendas. Beliefs and hidden agendas strongly influence a person's response to anxiety. For example, a lonely parent may be as ambivalent about a child's going to school as is the youngster. The parent then subtly reinforces "school refusal" behavior. A client who is easily threatened and needs to control the lives of his or her family may be content to do all the work for an agoraphobic spouse. Recognizing that change in one part of the family brings change for each member, the family therapist can assess for individual responses as well as the interaction between family members regarding the client's anxiety.

Many of the guidelines used for treating depression also hold true for treating anxious clients and their families. In addition, current research and information about anxiety disorders provide several clinical guidelines for working with anxious clients and their families:

- For panic disorders and phobias, consider cognitive-behavioral treatments.
- Consider the role family or marital conflict has in influencing the member's anxious symptoms.
- Consider covert or hidden relational interactions that influence the member's anxious symptoms (e.g., the partner's need to control or "protect" the anxious member).
- Consider the place or function of the anxious symptoms in the family system and the marital system.
- When treating anxious children, evaluate how the parents cope with stress and what coping skills they have taught their children.

ALCOHOLISM AND DRUG ABUSE

Substance abuse, whether it involves alcohol, illegal drugs, or prescribed medication, can occur when the therapist least expects it. Unless the therapist works at a drug and alcohol treatment center, few couples or families identify substance abuse as the presenting problem—exactly the opposite usually occurs. The family presents because a child is acting out in school and the school has required therapy for behavior problems. A couple requests marital therapy after years of tension and the wife's recent ultimatum, and the therapist begins treatment only to discover a substance abuse problem.

Individual therapists can simply ask the patient about substance use, but a family therapist may have to search for the abuse before it becomes apparent. The family may be so used to the abuser's behavior that it no longer considers it a problem, at least overtly. Family members may be frightened, ashamed, or intimidated into denying (at least verbally to an outsider) that there is a substance abuse problem. They can only get to therapy by requesting help for something else. The most important advice for a beginning family therapist is this: Consider the possibility of a substance abuse problem during your assessment, regardless of the presenting problems, and reconsider the possibility every time a constellation of symptoms, explanations, or descriptions does not make sense. Table 9.4 provides a quick reference for DSM-IV-TR diagnostic criteria for substance dependence and abuse.

The professional debates surrounding substance abuse can be confusing to a new therapist who is trying to learn the basics. Current controversies surround the issues of whether an alcoholic can ever drink again, whether alcoholism is a biological disease, whether recreational drug use leads to abuse and addiction, whether an "addictive personality" exists, and whether this personality develops from childhood trauma. Diagnosis is further confused by the arbitrary distinctions made between use, abuse, and dependence.

The beginning family therapist might consider these ongoing controversies intellectually interesting. However, for the therapist developing basic clinical skills, these arguments can distract from the primary goal—to get the person to stop using or abusing the substance. One therapist explained the goal of substance abuse work by comparing it to surgery: "I simply want to cut the harmful substance out of the person's life and then I'll do a pathology summary later, when the person is no longer being harmed." Substance abusers, family members, and other professionals can get caught up in myriad debates surrounding substance abuse and never focus on the simple behavioral issue of stopping the problem.

TABLE 9.4. Quick Reference for Substance Dependence and Substance Abuse

Criteria for substance dependence[a]

A maladaptive pattern of substance use, leading to clinically significant impairment or distress, as manifested by three (or more) of the following, occurring at any time in the same 12-month period:

(1) tolerance, as defined by either of the following:
   (a) a need for markedly increased amounts of the substance to achieve intoxication or desired effect
   (b) markedly diminished effect with continued use of the same amount of the substance
(2) withdrawal, as manifested by either of the following:
   (a) the characteristic withdrawal syndrome for the substance (refer to DSM-IV-TR criteria sets for withdrawal from specific substances)
   (b) the same (or a closely related) substance is taken to relieve or avoid withdrawal symptoms
(3) the substance is often taken in larger amounts or over a longer period than was intended
(4) there is a persistent desire or unsuccessful efforts to cut down or control substance use
(5) a great deal of time is spent in activities necessary to obtain the substance (e.g., visiting multiple doctors or driving long distances), use the substance (e.g., chain-smoking), or recover from its effects
(6) important social, occupational, or recreational activities are given up or reduced because of substance use
(7) the substance use is continued despite knowledge of having a persistent or recurrent physical or psychological problem that is likely to have been caused or exacerbated by the substance (e.g., current cocaine use despite recognition of cocaine-induced depression, or continued drinking despite recognition that an ulcer was made worse by alcohol consumption)

Criteria for substance abuse[b]

A. A maladaptive pattern of substance use leading to clinically significant impairment or distress, as manifested by one (or more) of the following, occurring within a 12-month period:
   (1) recurrent substance use resulting in a failure to fulfill major role obligations at work, school, or home (e.g., repeated absences or poor work performance related to substance use; substance-related absences, suspensions, or expulsions from school; neglect of children or household)
   (2) recurrent substance use in situations in which it is physically hazardous (e.g., driving an automobile or operating a machine when impaired by substance use)
   (3) recurrent substance-related legal problems (e.g., arrests for substance-related disorderly conduct)
   (4) continued substance use despite having persistent or recurrent social or interpersonal problems caused or exacerbated by the effects of the substance (e.g., arguments with spouse about consequences of intoxication, physical fights)

B. The symptoms have never met the criteria for substance dependence for this class of substance.

[a]See DSM-IV-TR for various specifiers. From American Psychiatric Association (2000, p. 197). Copyright 2000 by the American Psychiatric Association. Reprinted by permission.
[b]From American Psychiatric Association (2000, p. 199). Copyright 2000 by the American Psychiatric Association. Reprinted by permission.

Substance abuse is much more common in men than women. As a result, behaviors that reflect lapses in judgment and reasoning and lack of control, such as violence and sexual abuse, are much more common in men. If a family therapist scratches the surface of many deviant social behaviors committed by men, he or she will usually find comorbid substance abuse.

Substance abuse is a serious and common problem in the United States, and is related to drunk driving, suicide, homicide, violent crime, child and spouse abuse, and "household accidents." In addition, the biological effects of substance abuse, including cirrhosis, hepatitis, and seizures, can permanently damage a person's health. Alcoholism can be a true systemic illness—fetal alcohol syndrome is one of the only illnesses in which the mother is responsible for the damaging behavior and the child feels the effects, forever.

Assessments of alcoholism and substance abuse have been addressed in an earlier chapter. The purpose here is to review clinical and research literature that examines the role of alcoholism in the family and effective family treatments. Alcoholism and substance abuse are among the DSM-IV-TR categories that have received the most investigation by family therapists, perhaps because of evidence that alcoholism and substance abuse are "family diseases" in the sense that the abuser's behavior affects everyone in the family and, in turn, the abuser is affected by family members. Thus, many treatment programs involve family members and view interventions into family interaction as part of the treatment. For example, a goal of behavioral couples therapy is to increase relationship factors that are conducive to abstinence (O'Farrell & Fals-Stewart, 2006).

Research on alcoholic families suggests that a family's rituals, routines, and beliefs are strongly influenced by alcohol. In essence, the family can take on an "alcoholic identity" and collude to allow the alcoholic behavior to continue. At times, positive effects of the alcohol, not just damaging effects, are experienced by the family. For example, a family may be reluctant to encourage a husband and father who is more relaxed and engaging when he drinks to stop the drinking.

Some researchers take a developmental view of substance abuse. They suggest that seeds of an alcoholic family identity are planted early in the marriage, as a couple decides on patterns to follow and beliefs to hold—largely an implicit process (Steinglass, Bennett, Wolin, & Reiss, 1987). The role of alcohol and drinking in the family, while influenced by family of origin patterns, is one of the "decisions" a new couple makes. In essence, several small "agreements" to accept alcohol and alcoholic behavior can lead to a big "yes," and an alcoholic family is formed.

We believe that every alcoholic family must contend with the following characteristics of alcoholism: It is chronic; it involves use of a psychobiologically active drug; it is cyclical in nature; it produces predictable behavioral responses; and it has a definite course of development. However, families are more diverse than they are alike in their responses to these issues, and the role of alcohol must be assessed for each individual family.

Recent research reviews and meta-analyses of alcohol and drug studies have examined the efficacy of different psychosocial interventions (Dutra et al., 2008). Psychosocial treatments evaluated included contingency management, relapse prevention, cognitive-behavioral therapy, and other combined treatments. In general, contingency management, a system of rewards and punishments for specific behaviors, proved the most effective. Motivational interviewing, a treatment that focuses on understanding the client's level of motivation, has proven effective also (Arkowitz, Weston, Miller, & Rellnick, 2008). Principles from these models can be applied in a family format.

Specific situations might influence the efficacy of family treatments for alcoholism (Edwards & Steinglass, 1995; O'Farrell & Fals-Stewart, 2006; Rowe & Liddle, 2007). Families have a strong influence in motivating alcoholics to get treatment and to alter their drinking behavior. Family involvement, especially inclusion of nonalcoholic family members in the assessment phase, can be a routine component of alcoholism treatment. The impact of family treatment seems to vary according to gender (it is more helpful for men than for women to have spouses involved), investment in the relationship (an investment here produces greater motivation to change drinking behaviors), and support for abstinence from the family.

Most of these studies had control groups and several types of treatment groups. They generally found family therapy to be as effective as or more effective than other treatments. Family therapy was almost always superior to no-treatment control groups. Research suggests that involving the nonalcoholic spouse in treatment significantly improves outcome and can lead to more abstinence, happier relationships, less domestic violence, and fewer marital separations (Jacobson & Gurman, 1995; O'Farrell & Fals-Stewart, 2006). In addition, children can benefit from family-based treatments for substance problems.

Interestingly, many successful drug treatment programs derive from a structural/strategic tradition, while effective alcohol treatment programs derive from a behavioral therapy tradition (Fals-Stewart, O'Farrell, Birchler, Cordova, & Kelley, 2005; Rowe & Liddle, 2007). Both of these theoretical approaches share an active, problem-solving method with a focus on the present situation. Facilitating communication and problem-solving skills among family members is a key element of these treatments. While there is still much to be learned about treating substance abuse problems and alcoholism with family therapy, one can conclude that an active, focused style is essential for effectiveness.

Beginning clinicians often ask, "Is family therapy or marital therapy enough, or should it be used in conjunction with other forms of treatment?" The answer depends on the specific circumstances of the family. Many family therapy treatments are combined with individual treatments, education programs, and pharmacological treatment. In general, research shows that behavioral couple therapy produces greater abstinence and better relationship functioning than typical individual-based treatments alone. For many patients with the necessary resources, a combined treatment approach may be ideal.

Some family therapy programs combine aspects of other therapies into the family approach. For example, Liddle uses an individual therapist to form an alliance with substance-abusing adolescents and a separate family therapist to do the family treatment (Liddle & Dakof, 1995; Rowe & Liddle, 2007). One way to decide whether family therapy should be the sole treatment is to assess the intensity of the family's impact on the problem. For example, family therapy is more effective than other treatments for younger teens but not to the same degree for older teens (Sprenkle & Bischoff, 1991). In addition, behavioral marital therapy or spouse involvement in treatment for alcoholism is more effective for couples who report some marital distress before treatment. The old adage "If it ain't broke, don't fix it" comes to mind. Some research, however, suggests that even couples without marital distress see improved marital satisfaction and communication skills, and prevent deterioration of the relationship, when marital therapy is used to treat substance abuse (Alexander, Holtzworth-Munroe, & Jameson, 1994; O'Farrell & Fals-Stewart, 2006).

In determining whether marital or family therapies should be the sole treatment for a substance problem, the therapist can ask the abuser how much he or she would like the family to participate. On the other hand, limited resources or a structured treatment program may make this decision moot. In general, marital and family therapy should make up part of the treatment, given the growing evidence of its effectiveness.

Another benefit of including family therapy, besides ameliorating the substance abuse, is improvement in family members' satisfaction with marital and family relationships. When treatment ends, the family has a shared experience and new beliefs to refer back to in times of stress. The spouse can provide reminders of the benefits of the treatment several years after it is over. The potential effects of spouse and family involvement, even when the IP has a substance problem, are noted in the superior follow-up results of family therapy groups compared to other treatment groups.

If the goal is lasting change, not just a quick fix, it makes sense to include the most important people in the abuser's life in treatment because family members will still be with the patient long after therapy has ended. Literature on alcoholism and substance abuse suggests the following clinical guidelines:

- Regardless of the presenting problem, consider the possibility and role of substance abuse.
- Assess the role of alcohol or the substance in the family. For example, one family reported that their father was "the most fun and relaxed" when he was drinking, and thus the family saw the drinking as serving some positive functions for them.
- Consider the possibility of "enabling behaviors" by other family members.
- Assess how pervasive the substance is in influencing family beliefs, rituals, and routines.
- Accept that various family members will have different views on the seriousness of the substance problem. Some members may minimize the problem and others may focus on the substance use as the key problem in the family.
- Consider the possibility of violence or abuse occurring in the family because they are frequently comorbid with substance use.
- Consider stopping family therapy and refocusing treatment on stopping the member's substance abuse.

IMPULSE CONTROL DISORDERS

Recent research suggests that mental health specialists have overlooked the frequency of impulse control disorders, which generally refer to the following DSM diagnoses: oppositional defiant disorder, conduct disorder, intermittent explosive disorder, and the most well-known disorder in this category, attention-deficit/hyperactivity disorder (Dell'Osso, Marazziti, Hollander, & Altamura, 2007; Grant, 2008). These disorders are much more common than had been realized in earlier years, and are not confined to active schoolboys who can't sit in their chairs. Instead, these problems can be lifelong and share a common feature—struggles with emotional dysregulation (Gross,

2007). Unfortunately, within the group of most commonly occurring problems, impulse problems are most likely to be overlooked and undertreated. In addition, impulse problems most frequently occur in males, not females, and men are much less likely to seek treatment than women. If schools do not help identify children with impulse problems, the next public institution to address their struggles is often the legal system.

Oppositional defiant disorder and conduct disorder are usually diagnosed in childhood or late adolescence. Both refer to behavior problems, usually in boys (see Table 9.5). Oppositional defiant disorder is less serious than conduct disorder. Most of these problems initially manifest in the home and then appear in other settings such as schools. In fact, research correlates certain qualities of the home environment with the occurrence of these problems. For example, oppositional defiant disorder is commonly found in children growing up in homes with serious marital discord. Children with ADHD often grow up in homes where drug or alcohol dependence by one or both parents is an issue. Other research suggests that large family size, poor mental health of the mother, a father who has a criminal record, and high family conflict all correlate with the presence of impulse control disorders in children. Studies have also found that impulse disorders run in families, often because of genetic links. Thus, ample opportunities exist for a family therapist to intervene and help families and patients whose lives go awry because of these disorders.

While a boy's impulse problems may be more visible than a girl's internalizing depression, they are still frequently ignored or not treated. In addition, when children with unrecognized ADHD grow up, it is highly unlikely that they will ever be diagnosed and treated. This is in spite of good evidence suggesting the deleterious effects of ADHD and impulse control disorders in general. While we know that adult ADHD is associated with loss of jobs, families, and income and a host of other negative effects, usually the patient is blamed for his "personal failings" (Kessler et al., 2006). In fact, research suggests the correlates of adult ADHD include being divorced and unemployed.

Most impulse problems start at a young age (Pallanti, 2006). In fact, parents often report that they cannot remember a time when their child's behavior was not impulsive. However, recent neuroscience findings suggest that children who have behavior problems at young ages are not doomed to lives of failure. In fact, the origins of at least some types of ADHD indicate delays in brain development, not a learning deficit. And these young brains often catch up, especially with a supportive, healthy home and school environment.

TABLE 9.5. Quick Reference for Impulse Control Disorders

Disorder	Description
Attention-deficit/ hyperactivity disorder	Characterized by prominent symptoms of inattention and/or hyperactivity–impulsivity, and lack of emotion regulation.
Conduct disorder	Characterized by a pattern of behavior that violates the basic rights of others or major age-appropriate societal norms or rules.
Oppositional defiant disorder	Characterized by a pattern of negativistic, hostile, and defiant behavior.

Criteria for attention-deficit/hyperactivity disorder[a]

A. Either (1) or (2):

   (1) six (or more) of the following symptoms of **inattention** have persisted for at least 6 months to a degree that is maladaptive and inconsistent with developmental level:

Inattention
   (a) often fails to give close attention to details or makes careless mistakes in schoolwork, work, or other activities
   (b) often has difficulty sustaining attention in tasks or play activities
   (c) often does not seem to listen when spoken to directly
   (d) often does not follow through on instructions and fails to finish schoolwork, chores, or duties in the workplace (not due to oppositional behavior or failure to understand instructions)
   (e) often has difficulty organizing tasks and activities
   (f) often avoids, dislikes, or is reluctant to engage in tasks that require sustained mental effort (such as schoolwork or homework)
   (g) often loses things necessary for tasks or activities (e.g., toys, school assignments, pencils, books, or tools)
   (h) is often easily distracted by extraneous stimuli
   (i) is often forgetful in daily activities

   (2) six (or more) of the following symptoms of **hyperactivity–impulsivity** have persisted for at least 6 months to a degree that is maladaptive and inconsistent with developmental level:

Hyperactivity
   (a) often fidgets with hands or feet or squirms in seat
   (b) often leaves seat in classroom or in other situations in which remaining seated is expected
   (c) often runs about or climbs excessively in situations in which it is inappropriate (in adolescents or adults, may be limited to subjective feelings of restlessness)
   (d) often has difficulty playing or engaging in leisure activities quietly
   (e) is often "on the go" or often acts as if "driven by a motor"
   (f) often talks excessively

(cont.)

TABLE 9.5. *(cont.)*

Impulsivity
(g) often blurts out answers before questions have been completed
(h) often has difficulty awaiting turn
(i) often interrupts or intrudes on others (e.g., butts into conversations or games)

B. Some hyperactive-impulsive or inattentive symptoms that caused impairment were present before age 7 years.

C. Some impairment from the symptoms is present in two or more settings (e.g., at school [or work] and at home).

D. There must be clear evidence of clinically significant impairment in social, academic, or occupational functioning.

E. The symptoms do not occur exclusively during the course of a pervasive developmental disorder, schizophrenia, or other psychotic disorder and are not better accounted for by another mental disorder (e.g., mood disorder, anxiety disorder, dissociative disorder, or a personality disorder).

Criteria for conduct disorder[b]

A. A repetitive and persistent pattern of behavior in which the basic rights of others or major age-appropriate societal norms or rules are violated, as manifested by the presence of three (or more) of the following criteria in the past 12 months, with at least one criterion present in the past 6 months:

Aggression toward people and animals
(1) often bullies, threatens, or intimidates others
(2) often initiates physical fights
(3) has used a weapon that can cause serious physical harm to others (e.g., a bat, brick, broken bottle, knife, gun)
(4) has been physically cruel to people
(5) has been physically cruel to animals
(6) has stolen while confronting a victim (e.g., mugging, purse snatching, extortion, armed robbery)
(7) has forced someone into sexual activity

Destruction of property
(8) has deliberately engaged in fire setting with the intention of causing serious damage
(9) has deliberately destroyed others' property (other than by setting fire)

Deceitfulness or theft
(10) has broken into someone else's house, building, or car
(11) often lies to obtain goods or favors or to avoid obligations (i.e., "cons" others)
(12) has stolen items of nontrivial value without confronting a victim (e.g., shoplifting, but without breaking and entering; forgery)

(cont.)

TABLE 9.5. *(cont.)*

Serious violations of rules
(13) often stays out at night despite parental prohibitions, beginning before age 13 years
(14) has run away from home overnight at least twice while living in parental or parental surrogate home (or once without returning for a lengthy period)
(15) is often truant from school, beginning before age 13 years

B. The disturbance in behavior causes clinically significant impairment in social, academic, or occupational functioning.

C. If the individual is 18 years or older, criteria are not met for antisocial personality disorder.

Criteria for oppositional defiant disorder[c]

A. A pattern of negativistic, hostile, and defiant behavior lasting at least 6 months, during which four (or more) of the following are present:

(1) often loses temper
(2) often argues with adults
(3) often actively defies or refuses to comply with adults' requests or rules
(4) often deliberately annoys people
(5) often blames others for his or her mistakes or misbehavior
(6) is often touchy or easily annoyed by others
(7) is often angry and resentful
(8) is often spiteful or vindictive

B. The disturbance in behavior causes clinically significant impairment in social, academic, or occupational functioning.

C. The behaviors do not occur exclusively during the course of a psychotic or mood disorder.

D. Criteria are not met for conduct disorder, and, if the individual is 18 years or older, criteria are not met for antisocial personality disorder.

[a]From American Psychiatric Association (2000, p. 92). Copyright 2000 by the American Psychiatric Association. Reprinted by permission.
[b]From American Psychiatric Association (2000, pp. 98–99). Copyright 2000 by the American Psychiatric Association. Reprinted by permission.
[c]From American Psychiatric Association (2000, p. 102). Copyright 2000 by the American Psychiatric Association. Reprinted by permission.

Impulse control problems are an area where family therapists can make a big difference if they are identified before a child reaches adulthood. But even this process can be challenging. For girls, impulse control problems might manifest in aggression toward other girls and be ignored by adults as "teenage angst." Girls with attention problems are often daydreamers, rather than hyperactive, and poor academic performance can be attributed to lack of motivation. Thus, many girls with impulse problems are never diagnosed. In addition, once a young person reaches adulthood, his or her learning style is often set and employment struggles or other deficits are attributed to "laziness" or "lack of motivation." Even if the child's problems are correctly identified, parents are often reluctant to consider medication, the mainstay of treatment for ADHD.

Impulse problems are often connected to underlying emotions such as anger or aggressive feelings. ADHD has a core group of symptoms including impulsivity, inattention, emotional dysregulation problems, and motor restlessness. Oppositional defiant disorder has core symptoms such as defiance and hostility, while conduct disorder can be characterized by willful disregard for the rights of others and includes behaviors such as cruelty, destruction of property, lying, and theft. Even if impulse problems don't lead to criminal behavior, the symptoms can still lead to an adult life of frustration, anger, and failure.

Family therapists can make a significant difference in helping families that struggle with impulse problems. Besides considering medication for at least some diagnoses, such as ADHD, family therapists can focus on emotion regulation in the family. How are frustration, anger, and disappointment handled in the family? Often, parents with their own emotional struggles, such as a depressed mother or a violent father, will overrespond or underrespond to their children's needs for soothing, emotional validation, and structure. These patterns often start early, when the child is an infant, and continue to adulthood.

If parents have the emotional resources and ability to help their children, research suggests that parental soothing and structuring can make a difference by helping children learn how to identify their feelings, master their behaviors, and calm themselves down. In turn, these abilities can lead to lifelong skills in "executive functioning"—being able to organize one's life and cope with stress. In general, the earlier parents get started on addressing both their own emotional struggles and their children's challenges, the easier the task. Family therapists can serve as coaches and consultants to parents—giving them the information and tools they need to create a home environment where children can prosper. In addition, family therapists can help parents advocate for their children's needs in school systems and try to ensure that the learning environment is optimal. Family therapists should be familiar with the laws and policies that guarantee children access to resources for neuropsychological testing and other assessment measures. They can help the family obtain an individualized educational plan (IEP) for the child.

However, if impulse control disorders remain undiagnosed, problems persist into adulthood. Family therapists can look for patterns of loss and failure in their adult patients that initially seem unexplained. Frequent job changes, incomplete educations, disrupted relationships, poor driving records, and histories of substance abuse are all warning signs that the patient may suffer from an impulse disorder. Often, instead of feeling stigmatized by a diagnostic label, patients feel relief when they are finally given an explanation for their painful history. As one patient said, "I'm so glad there is a name for what I have because before now the only name I had for it was 'loser.'"

Research shows that some small changes early in a child's life can have a significant effect as the child ages. Thinking in simple cost-benefit terms, it makes sense to help parents with their own issues and then to help them parent effectively. In fact, a major study documenting the presence of mental disorders beginning at early ages suggests that public health interventions should be more focused on children and adolescence (Kessler et al., 2005). With these ideas in mind, family therapists can consider the following goals when working with families with impulse struggles:

- When you are treating a child or teen for impulse problems, expand your assessment to the parents. Both genetic and environmental influences often lead to multiple family members struggling with control of their impulses.
- Make sure you are up to date on the literature, especially for ADHD, and make psychoeducation a significant part of your treatment.
- Work with the family on both behavioral interventions for creating structure and emotional interventions for creating soothing and self-regulation.
- Involve other systems such as the schools, and teach the parents how to advocate for their children.
- Use outside resources. Consider neuropsychological testing, psychotropic medication, tutoring and coaching, and other measures to help the family.

CONCLUSION

Alcoholism or drug abuse, anxiety, impulse struggles, and depression are four of the most common individual disorders a therapist will encounter in clinical practice. A therapist must not view these disorders in a vacuum but rather within the context of existing and past social and emotional problems and the family's extant strengths and weaknesses. In addition, a therapist must keep in mind that the family of an individual with a mental disorder is often inextricably involved in the perpetuation or containment of this disorder and that psychoeducation and support are crucial to the well-being of the whole family as well as that of their afflicted member.

CHAPTER 10

Getting Unstuck in Therapy

"I've been working with this family for several weeks, but not much seems to be changing. Now what do I do?" Supervisors and seasoned colleagues often hear this question from beginning therapists. Clearly, therapy is not always a smooth ride for any of its participants, and therapists frequently encounter a multitude of complications and obstacles along the way. Consider the case of the Smith family:

The Smiths initially presented their 16-year-old daughter's sexual acting out as their primary problem. A letter had been discovered by her mother detailing her sexual fantasies and possible encounters with a young man who lived a few hundred miles away. The family sessions included two teenage daughters, ages 16 and 13, and the parents. The family—bright, verbal, and well educated—could express its ideas well, but had considerable difficulty with direct communication and expression of feelings. After several family sessions, the family stabilized and everyone agreed that many of the difficulties were the result of long-standing marital problems.

Couple therapy began as a slow and painful process for the spouses in this family. Considerable sexual tension, a lack of feeling disclosure, and a history of fighting culminated in hurt feelings and emotional withdrawal. The husband had a history of going into rages in which he couldn't control his emotions and would break things in the house. These incidents, described by his wife as "childlike temper tantrums," resulted in the wife withdrawing, becoming depressed, and locking herself in her bedroom. Both individuals harbored a great deal of resentment for past unresolved conflicts dating back to their courtship. The husband insisted that the problem was essentially the wife's. His contention was that her withdrawal and lack of affection caused most of the difficulties. There was no evidence of alcohol abuse. The wife had taken antidepressants on several occasions. These were pre-scribed by her family doctor—she refused to see a psychiatrist.

The couple therapy progressed for several weeks with little change. The wife refused to talk about her family of origin issues, other than to say she was abused. She indicated that she felt her husband wouldn't understand and would only use the information against her. The hus-band was willing to discuss his family of origin, but saw little relevance in it for his marriage. The husband's frustration with the lack of contact and change increased. The wife's depressive symptoms intensified, and included crying spells, sleep problems, withdrawal, excessive worry-ing, and lethargy. She felt that the marital sessions were "too much" and were creating more stress and difficulty. The husband threatened divorce if his wife didn't change.

Family therapists expect people to be ambivalent about change. The struggle for change is inevitable within any relationship context, including the therapy room. The challenge of facilitating new ways and ending old ways is central to all therapeutic processes. In the following sections, we identify common sources of "stuckness" in therapy and provide options for thinking about and dealing with them.

UNDERSTANDING CLIENTS' AMBIVALENCE ABOUT CHANGE

Beginning therapists need to recognize that all clients have some ambivalence about change. Fortunately, the fact that clients even come into therapy usually shows some willingness to try something new or to apply energy in a different way. Further, the therapist's very partici-pation with a client or family can produce and promote change. True change, however, might not be welcomed by the people requesting it. All people have a tendency to go back to the ways things have always been done—homeostasis. Familiar is comfortable.

Resistance is a normal part of therapy, not an exception. Younger therapists sometimes think they have failed when they encounter resis-tance. In order to talk intelligently about client resistance, we need a definition. For resistance, we use the working definition offered in the excellent text *Mastering Resistance,* by Anderson and Stewart (1983), which states:

> Resistance can be defined as all those behaviors in the therapeutic system which interact to prevent the therapeutic system from achieving the fam-ily's goals for therapy. The therapeutic system includes all family mem-bers, the therapist, and the context in which the therapy takes place, that

is, the agency or institution in which it occurs. Resistance is most likely to be successful, that is, to result in the termination or failure of family therapy, when resistances are present and interacting synergistically in all three components of the therapeutic system. (p. 24)

Various theoretical orientations label clients' ambivalence about change and their resistance differently. For example, structural family therapy would find resistance in the family's failure to accommodate its structure to the changing developmental needs of its members, while transgenerational family therapies might assess resistance as an integral part of dealing with unfinished business in one's family of origin. Resistance in either case is a predictable partner of change. By definition then, a family therapist must clearly keep in mind both a theoretical approach as well as the family's goals for therapy in order to interpret resistance accurately. Resistance comes with the territory of therapy and must not be viewed as failure, but as an expected aspect of the work.

The client system fears change since it is something new and unpredictable. For example, a client might be an alcoholic, single mother who is coming into therapy because of her child's school problems. If the mother fails to look at the possible influence of her drinking (an examination usually carried out later in the therapeutic relationship) on the child's school problems, we have resistance. A client system might also be a couple in marital therapy that continues to practice abusive interactions between sessions, even though alternative interactions have been offered and practiced in therapy. Changing old and comfortable coping and communication patterns is threatening. The future is unknown to the client.

The therapist can provide significant emotional support to the client by recognizing ambivalence. Verbally acknowledging that change is hard, scary, and uncomfortable helps. Also, giving the resistance "back to the client" is an important method of diffusing rather than escalating resistance. Telling the client, "You're changing too much" or "You're proceeding too fast" or "There must be other, more important concerns that keep you from trying new things" or "Maybe the old way wasn't so bad after all" drops the pressure from the therapist and allows the client to reevaluate the desired area for growth.

THE THERAPIST'S RELUCTANCE TO INTERVENE

Many normal obstacles interfere with successful therapy, especially in the beginning. Central to removing these barriers is a willingness to learn from one's mistakes and be open to information. Supportive, safe, and "live data" supervision (using videotape or cotherapy) offers vital information in helping beginning therapists avoid problems and find a solid footing.

The rules of therapy are different from those in polite conversation. What might seem like interrupting someone in casual discourse may be an intervention in therapy. Some clients will talk continuously with a lack of clarity. The therapist may need to intervene in order to help them refocus or keep them on track. In intervening, the therapist is looking for an opening to redirect the client and maintain continuity.

Sometimes trainees do not risk an intervention until everything is totally clear. Lack of experience and anxiety over dealing with presenting issues can result in gathering too much information or spending many sessions unfocused. Clients need to experience some progress early in the therapy—without this, they might not come back. One idea is to offer some therapeutic "gift" to the client early, even before the direction of therapy has been decided. These gifts include interventions such as normalizing, reframing, amplifying positive interactions in the family, or congratulating the family on their courage to seek help.

Also, after two to three sessions, the therapist may want to use the clinical reasoning process discussed in Chapter 5 to understand the presenting problems and to focus on possible interventions. Once this is done, you just need to jump in and risk trying something.

THERAPIST–CLIENT AGENDA AND TIMING MISMATCH

Another key area of "stuckness" comes from a mismatch between the therapist's goals and the family's goals. Especially enthusiastic at the start of their work, family therapy practicum students often want to "change the world" and "fix" the family. The therapist–client mismatch becomes particularly clear when a therapist begins to direct the family toward something they don't want. For example, a 10-year-old child of a single mother is brought to therapy because of chronic lying at school and at home. The therapist focuses on the task of involving the father, who has visited with the child only five times in her life, in solving the problem, and the mother doesn't return to therapy. When a therapist focuses more on a theoretical perspective or his or her own agenda than the working relationship with the client, a mismatch is more likely to occur.

Change can be achieved at different levels, referred to as first-order and second-order change. First-order change denotes behavioral change, that is, acting in new ways. Second-order change requires behavioral, cognitive, affective, and relational changes, that is, change within an entire system. It's important to determine what order of change the therapist and client systems desire so that therapy is planned appropriately. Usually, struggles occur around the systemic differences in defining the "right kind of change." For example, a rigid, authoritarian parent may present his son for therapy because of problems with homework. After focusing on this presenting problem by bringing some flexibility into when and where the child does the homework, the parent terminates therapy. The therapist, however, wants to address the overall rigidity of the parental system during adolescence and wants to continue therapy to achieve more adaptability—for the entire family, and for the son's future growth. The parent requests first-order change, which is at odds with the therapist's desire to generate second-order change. The following case further illustrates the differences between these levels of change.

A 15-year-old girl is presented as the IP in her family. The current problem is her continuing to come home late in the evening, after her imposed curfew. The parents have attempted to change her behavior by first simply asking that she come home on time or call. The girl agreed, but continued to come home late. The parents then told her that if she was late one night, she would have to come home early the next night by the same amount of time. She agreed to try this but later said it was unfair, and that their curfew was too early to begin with.

In the therapy session, the parents were asked to talk about their concerns and feelings for their daughter. They also talked about their fears of her growing up and leaving them, and of their lack of contact with her friends. At one point the father said, "I just feel like I don't know who you are anymore." The girl disclosed some of her frustrations with her parents and some of the pressures she was under at school.

Although the problems were not immediately solved, the parents and their daughter were able to talk about their stresses and feelings about change in their relationship. They worked out a new approach to the problem of coming home late by discussing their individual perspectives on the problem and several possible solutions.

The parents' attempts to change the situation before coming to therapy were primarily aimed at changing the girl's behavior. First, they asked her to come home on time and then they tried to develop consequences for not coming in on time. These are examples of first-order change that is targeted at the behavioral level. In the therapy session, family members explored their relationships and feelings about each other. They also discussed concerns about the problem and about the changes they were facing. Ultimately, the changes that began to take place in the family's ability to communicate moved beyond behaviors. Changes slowly occurred on several levels, including the affective, relational, and behavioral domains, which would impact the entire family system. Thus, we have second-order change.

In addition to being clear about the level of change desired by client and therapist, timing of interventions must be considered. Family therapy highlights the need to be intentional about when certain tasks need to be done and who needs to be a part of the change. This concern is revisited throughout therapy. A remarried couple might need to solve differences and work on better communication skills before inviting an ex-wife to join in sessions concerning a college-age daughter. If the ex-wife was brought in before the remarried couple dealt with their own conflicts, a therapist might see resistance. The therapist must handle the important issues of matching agendas and timing to proceed effectively.

THERAPISTS' LACK OF THEORETICAL CLARITY

Another common therapist contribution to problems in the therapeutic process stems from a lack of clarity about one's theoretical perspective. Beginning therapists jump at the opportunity to translate what they've learned in class into a counseling session. After joining and assessment, the therapist might take a grab-bag approach to interventions. For example, John and Jean enter therapy after an argument in which they decide to call off their engagement. As high school sweethearts, they and their fairly enmeshed families have found increasing tension around wedding plans—styles and expectations differ. A therapist begins to work on the couple's communication and problem-solving skills during the first two working sessions, but then shifts to a structural perspective in order to more appropriately separate a mother–daughter alignment. In a subsequent session, we find the therapist encouraging the expression of grief. While none of these clinical interventions or understandings is incorrect, the therapist might begin to lose focus on the theoretical perspective, appropriate interventions for that theory, and therapeutic goals. When this happens, supervisors often hear practicum students say, "I'm lost."

Your theoretical orientation helps to define what domain of therapy is central to your work with a particular client. Affective, behavioral, cognitive, and/or relational domains may be affected. It's important for the therapist to keep in mind which of these domains therapy will impact. For example, in experiential therapies the domain of affect needs to be emphasized. Thus, a therapist might have difficulty debriefing a family sculpture that depicts a child's feeling left out when the family is one that doesn't readily allow for expression of sad feelings. Experiential therapy also requires family members to be in the therapy room in order for authentic and honest self-disclosure to be accomplished. It would be insufficient to address being left out if the child was not present. In contrast, from a strategic perspective where behavioral sequences are central, the parents of an oppositional adolescent son might resist "catching their child following the rules" when he does follow them. The son wouldn't necessarily need to be in the room in order to facilitate change in this family.

Therapists who are focused and intentional about what they offer to a family will help clients manage their resistance positively. Therapists who lose focus about therapeutic goals and domains of therapy (as addressed by their theoretical orientation) will frustrate both themselves and their clients. This process can be complicated when new therapists receive conflicting feedback from different supervisors, each with different therapeutic agendas.

The most helpful way to stay on track in facilitating change is to set clear goals with the family during the first few sessions and then select theoretical perspectives that will best serve reaching those goals. A conscious blending of several theories is often appropriate; however, goals need to be prioritized—which are of first, second, or third importance? These issues should be handled by the therapist and family in the initial sessions at regular intervals. Without prioritizing the goals, session agendas are unclear for everyone.

SUPERVISION

Supervision can be one of the most important ways for you to get help on a case. Ideally, you will have access to a supervisor who has both strong clinical and supervisory skills. Individuals who are Approved Supervisors through the American Association for Marriage and Family Therapy (AAMFT), for example, have received special instruction in supervision (including supervision of their supervision) and have at least 2 years of postlicensure clinical experience.

Although the supervisor's qualifications are important, you must also be willing to do your part to make the supervision experience worthwhile. This requires that you be willing to share issues and cases that are a source of struggle for you. You need to be willing to seek live supervision or show videotapes of cases in which you feel stuck or frustrated. Therapists who only present cases in which they feel competent are missing an opportunity to grow and stretch themselves through supervision.

You must also be willing to give your supervisor feedback on what is needed from supervision. You might specify a particular issue you would like feedback on in a case, or you might indicate the need for more positive feedback if you are struggling with confidence issues. In some cases, you may need to tell your supervisor that the suggestions do not seem to fit the family, and explore with him or her why this is the case, which may lead to new, more helpful insights. Most supervisors will appreciate any feedback you can provide that gives a clearer sense of what is needed from supervision.

Although supervision is generally invaluable to beginning therapists, it can also present some challenges. If you are getting supervision from more than one person, you may receive different or conflicting advice on a case. In some cases you will be able to resolve the problem by listening to your clinical intuition. By virtue of spending a lot of time with your clients, you may have an intuitive feel as to which approach will offer the best fit. If you do not have an intuitive feeling as to which approach is best, then this may be a sign that further assessment is needed. Collecting additional information may help clarify which conceptualization is a better fit with the case. You may even consider presenting both perspectives to the clients, and ask for their feedback on which conceptualization is most valid or helpful. Finally, you might consider bringing the issue of conflicting advice back into supervision with one or both supervisors. Supervision can then explore the possible advantages and disadvantages of each approach, as well as possible ways to resolve the contradictory perspectives.

Therapists may encounter problems in supervision if there is not a good fit between the supervisor and therapist. "Goodness of fit" between therapist and supervisor can be determined by a number of factors. An issue of fit can arise if the supervisor and therapist conceptualize cases from different theoretical perspectives. Issues of fit can also arise out of a mismatch between the supervisor's approach and the therapist's needs. A therapist who is interested in exploring self-of-therapist issues in supervision, for example, may feel frustrated by a supervisor who focuses primarily on theory or conceptualizing cases. Supervisors can also differ in the extent to which they are directive or nondirective, hierarchical or collaborative, or in the balance between offering positive feedback and constructive feedback. These and other factors can influence the extent to which the therapist perceives the supervisor as a good fit with his or her needs. As stated above, you should be explicit in stating what you need from supervision, which will help the supervisor make the necessary adjustments to better meet your needs. If possible, you can also consider seeking additional supervision from others who may offer a better fit with your needs.

SELF-SUPERVISION QUESTIONS

In addition to getting supervision from a qualified supervisor, you should begin to develop your own self-supervision skills. In other words, you should develop self-reflective methods and questions that can be used in place of getting supervision from another individual. Watching videotapes of your own sessions is helpful in providing a more objective viewpoint on what happens in therapy. Often therapists who have watched their videotapes prior to receiving supervision will report gaining an important insight into their work.

You can also develop a list of self-supervision questions that are helpful when you get stuck in a case—a checklist of items that can frequently cause difficulties. A list of sample self-supervision questions is provided in Table 10.1. For example, a therapist who feels frustrated by the lack of movement in a case may discover upon going through the checklist of questions that he or she is working much harder than the clients. This in turn might lead the therapist to explore the clients' motivation for therapy or the possible negative consequences of change. Used in this manner, a checklist of questions can be an effective means of helping you troubleshoot a case on your own.

TABLE 10.1. Self-Supervision Questions

When feeling stuck or encountering client resistance, ask:

1. Am I, as the therapist, working harder than the clients?
2. What are negative consequences of change that my clients may be struggling with?
3. Does the problem serve some positive function or purpose?
4. Have I clearly assessed the client's goals, and does the client see me as working on those goals?
5. Have I sufficiently joined with the client?
6. Does the client see therapy or the therapist as credible?
7. Is my frustration a possible sign of my own personal issues interfering with the client's?
8. Are my reactions or responses isomorphic to the system?
9. Have I appropriately balanced the responsibility for change? (Or do I find myself siding with one client over another?)
10. Have I identified two or three key therapeutic issues or themes, or am I trying to focus on too many things?

DOING A LITERATURE SEARCH

The marriage and family therapy literature is a rich source of information for dealing with difficult cases. Reading the literature is particularly helpful in cases where you have limited experience with a particular problem or population. For example, a therapist who has not worked with a couple experiencing infertility could read books, research articles, or other literature on the issues that infertile couples must face.

The following six-step model (Williams, Patterson, & Miller, 2006) can be used to locate research or other literature to inform your clinical work. In Step 1, you need to define the purpose of your search. Are you primarily interested in issues of assessment, or are you looking for treatment approaches with regard to a case? Being more specific can help you narrow your search more efficiently.

After defining your purpose, you need to conduct a search to locate the pertinent literature (Step 2). PsycINFO (*www.apa.org/psycinfo*) offers the most comprehensive database of psychological research and literature, and is usually an excellent starting point. However, you may want to consider other databases. Evidence Based Mental Health (*ebmh. bmjjournals.com*), for example, is an online journal that summarizes mental health research from medical and psychiatry journals. Useful research may also be found by searching medical databases, particularly for issues related to health or psychopathology. Medline offers the most extensive listing of the biomedical literature, and can be accessed for free through PubMed (*www.ncbi.nlm.nih.gov/pubmed*). Highwire (*highwire.stanford.edu*) also offers free online access to many articles. Other databases like Cochrane Database of Systematic Reviews (*www. cochrane.org*), Clinical Evidence (*www.clinicalevidence.com*), Evidence Based Medicine (*ebm.bmjjournals.com*), and Evidence Based Medicine Reviews (*www.ovid.com*) can also be searched to locate relevant research from the medical field.

In Step 3, you will need to decide which research or literature you will obtain and read after doing your search. In most cases, the potential relevance of an article can be determined by scanning the title and abstract. Fortunately, it is becoming easier to access articles since many of them are available online. If an article is not easily available online, then you will have to weigh the cost or effort of obtaining the article against its potential relevance and usefulness.

In the fourth step, you will need to evaluate the quality of the research if the article summarizes an empirical study. Obviously, greater confidence can be placed in studies with stronger methodologies. Table 10.2 lists questions that a reader with a basic understanding

TABLE 10.2. Questions for Evaluating Research

Introduction and literature review

1. Are the purpose and importance of the study clearly articulated?
2. Does the literature review cover the relevant research?
3. Is the literature cited current?
4. Does the literature review critique the existing literature, or simply summarize it?

Methodology

Measurement issues
1. Are the instruments in the study adequately described?
2. Is there evidence of internal and/or test–retest reliability for measures used in the study?
3. Is there evidence for interrater reliability if coding systems are used?
4. Is there evidence that the instruments are valid (e.g., content, criterion, concurrent, and/or construct validity)?
5. Are there other measurement concerns (e.g., reactivity, sensitivity)?

Sampling issues and external validity
1. What steps were taken to make sure the sample was representative of the population of interest? Was probability (random, systematic, strata, multistage cluster) or nonprobability (e.g., convenience) sampling used?
2. Does a low response rate threaten the representativeness of the sample?
3. Are the demographics of the sample adequately described?
4. Does the sample adequately represent diversity (e.g., race/ethnicity, gender)?
5. Are the possible threats to generalizability (external validity) addressed in the research?

Issues of internal validity
1. For experimental studies, does the study include both a treatment and a comparison group (control or alternative treatment)? Are subjects randomly assigned to the groups?
2. Does the outcome study take into account possible confounding variables such as placebo effects, attention effects, or mortality rates?
3. Is there evidence that the treatments were delivered as intended, or that participants were compliant in following the treatment?
4. For correlational research, does the researcher inappropriately imply cause and effect relationships? Is there consideration of spurious relationships?
5. Are threats to internal validity from cohort effects addressed in cross-sectional research?

Methodological issues for qualitative research
1. Does the researcher identify the theoretical framework and other potential biases that may influence interpretation of the data?
2. Is the researcher role in relation to the participants clearly defined (e.g., participant vs. nonparticipant, concealed vs. nonconcealed)?
3. For qualitative research, were the criteria for selecting participants clearly described?
4. Does the researcher specify the types of data collected, and how they were collected?

(cont.)

TABLE 10.2. *(cont.)*

5. Does the researcher specify how the data were analyzed?
6. Does the researcher report how he or she established reliability and validity (e.g., triangulation of data, saturation, having participants examine the findings)?
7. Do the illustrative quotes or descriptions support the conclusions?

Other considerations
1. Are there any ethical concerns about the study (e.g., benefits outweigh risks, informed consent, voluntary, privacy)?
2. For outcome studies, are the treatments adequately described?
3. Were appropriate statistical tests used to analyze the findings?

Results and discussion

1. Does the researcher draw appropriate conclusions from the results, or do they go beyond what they should given the limits to the internal or external validity of the study?
2. Does the article clearly identify the limitations of the research?
3. Does the researcher address clinical significance or rely exclusively on statistical significance?
4. Are implications (or contraindications) for treatment discussed?
5. Are recommendations for future research included?

Note. From Williams, Patterson, and Miller (2006, pp. 31–32). Copyright 2006 by the American Association for Marriage and Family Therapy. Reprinted by permission.

of research can ask to discriminate studies that are generally strong from those with major weaknesses. However, more indirect measures of quality can also be used to evaluate the quality of research. Greater confidence can be put in studies that are in peer-reviewed journals. In addition, more prestigious journals typically have higher-quality studies since they can be more selective in the research they publish.

In most cases, you will be able to find multiple articles on the topic of interest. Therefore, in the fifth step you need to synthesize the information from the literature. Ideally, you will be able to identify some consistent trends or patterns, giving you greater confidence in the findings. As a possible shortcut, it is helpful to look for reviews of the literature or meta-analyses that conveniently summarize the research in an area rather than you having to do it.

In the sixth and final step, you will need to apply what you have learned from the literature to your case. You will first need to assess the extent to which the findings directly relate to the issue your client is addressing. In some cases, the literature may be directly relevant. In other cases, you may have to be more tentative in applying the findings since they do not directly relate to the issue. Second, you need to ask how similar your clients are to the ones who have been studied or described in the research. If they are different, then you will need to be more cautious in applying the findings to this particular case. In addition, you may need to make modifications taking into account differences such as culture, age, gender, sexual orientation, or other attributes. Third, additional steps may be necessary before you can successfully apply the research to the case, such as obtaining treatment manuals or assessment instruments from the authors.

In addition to using journal articles and books, therapists can also look up a lot of useful information on the Internet. However, if you use information from the Internet, you need to be certain the information is from a reliable source. Information from sites sponsored by organizations (e.g., universities, medical organizations) or the government are likely to be more reliable than sites created by individuals.

DEALING WITH CANCELLATIONS AND NO-SHOWS

A 19-year-old client who has been coming to therapy for depression missed an appointment because he had a job interview; he forgot to call the therapist and cancel the appointment. A younger adolescent client failed to make her morning appointment because she overslept, and she blamed her mother for not waking her up. A family being treated for anxiety in two children begins canceling and rescheduling appointments, and 4 weeks have gone by without a session.

Cancellations and missed appointments offer important information to the therapist and must be acknowledged and evaluated. Since systemic thinking assumes a relational nature to therapeutic work, cancellations and missed appointments need to be interpreted relationally. Therapists need to respond to both, usually by telephone, to determine the meaning of the no-show or cancellation. Sometimes the meaning is quite concrete and practical: It's simply a missed appointment—"I had a flat tire and couldn't get it fixed in time for our appointment." It's useful to review one's policy on cancellations and missed appointments at this time and to clarify any misunderstandings. Most agencies and practices have a 24-hour cancellation policy in which clients are billed for the appointment unless they cancel at least 24 hours before the appointment. This policy may be waived for emergencies; however, "emergency" must be defined.

No-shows or cancellations can indicate a reevaluation of the therapeutic process itself. Goals need to be evaluated throughout the therapeutic process, preferably with the clients' involvement. But when clients have difficulty with this, they might communicate their discomfort by canceling or missing appointments. For example, a couple comes to therapy to decrease the number of fights they have. This goal is partially addressed by encouraging solid communication skills such as "I" statements and active listening. After a bit of relief, the couple starts canceling or consistently rescheduling their appointments. The therapist requests a reevaluation session to discuss if therapy has satisfied the couple's goals and could be terminated, if appointments might be set at more infrequent intervals, or if other goals need to be addressed. It's important to set a collaborative tone for the reevaluation process since client and therapist goals might not match.

Cancellations and no-shows might also indicate that parts of the client system are questioning the therapeutic process. For example, as a depressed adolescent begins to speak more assertively about his needs, perhaps even yell sometimes, the rest of the family might wonder if therapy is doing any good, since this "isn't the behavior we wanted." Cancellations and missed appointments can simply indicate the system's ambivalence about change.

No-shows and cancellations might also result from a disruption in the therapeutic alliance. This is particularly true for clients with certain family of origin issues, such as abandonment, or with Axis II DSM-IV-TR diagnoses, such as borderline or avoidant personality disorders. Some clients might be extremely sensitive to a therapist's taking sides during a family session, experiencing the therapist's validation of another family member as invalidating them. Clients express this indirectly by not showing for an appointment or by "forgetting." Again, depending on the therapist's theoretical orientation, this aspect of the client's reaction will be explored in more or less depth. All therapists need to determine, on an ongoing basis, the solidity of the therapeutic alliance in order to proceed successfully in therapy.

Clients who lack significant motivation or stability in their lives are more likely to cancel or no show. Clients who are mandated to go to therapy can be expected to be sporadic in their attendance. Those who have been transferred from another therapist are also susceptible to missing appointments until they develop a relationship with the new therapist. Having realistic expectations regarding the client's level of motivation and desire for the therapy will help you manage your caseload more effectively.

Cancellations and missed appointments also result from practical constraints, especially for clients who are socially and economically disadvantaged. For example, a client may have to choose between paying for therapy and paying for groceries or rent. Also, lack of access to transportation can constrain one's ability to attend therapy. It's important to be sensitive to these realistic limitations and to negotiate ways of increasing resources to keep therapy accessible. There's nothing magic about scheduling therapy once a week. This format stems from early analytic patterns of scheduling three to five sessions each week. Systemic interventions can be creatively managed, as highlighted by the approach of some Italian family therapists (the Milan group), who might do several hours of intensive family work and then not see the family for several months.

The key is that the therapist participates actively in understanding the meaning of the no-show or cancellation and manages this meaning therapeutically.

DIFFICULTY GETTING OTHER FAMILY MEMBERS TO THERAPY

The family members who do not make it into treatment may be absent for several different reasons. The first area to investigate is communication between family members. Were they asked to be a part of therapy? How was this discussed? Sometimes therapy can be viewed as another issue to fight about, and it becomes the problem rather than a vehicle for solving problems. Each family member makes a choice in coming or not coming to therapy, exercising some power in the family's decision-making process. If a family member is involved in a power struggle, it may be helpful for the therapist to intervene as a mediator to invite the member to come to the session. Offering to make telephone contact with a reluctant client can serve as a bridge to therapy.

Family members may not come in because they don't think that they have a problem. It's not unusual for one member of a couple to want to go to therapy while the other is reluctant or ambivalent. The reluctant partner often feels that he or she does not really have a problem, so "why should I go?" It can be useful for the therapist to indicate to this partner that he or she has a valuable perspective and pertinent information to offer, regardless of who appears to have the problem. Further, the therapist might point out to reluctant clients that they are in the best position to relay their own story. Absence could mean their voice may go unheard or their position be misrepresented.

Some family members may be reluctant to attend sessions due to their discomfort with others in the family. In some situations, it may be useful to first work with subsystems and join effectively with them before bringing in all of the family members at once. In some families, being together and having direct communication is a rarity and may need to be "worked up to" on a gradual basis over several sessions.

Reluctant clients may be skeptical of the value of therapy or they may have had a previous negative experience in therapy. Their previous experiences and views about therapy should be explored and understood. It can be helpful to suggest that the client commit initially to only one visit. This session should provide an opportunity for the person to be heard as well as a chance for him or her to hear what other family members have to say. The focus of this session will likely be on providing a safe place for communication and not on making changes.

HANDLING SECRETS

Some therapists prefer the "clarity" of individual therapy, which simplifies the clinical contract. However, systemically oriented therapists understand that involving more than one person is a powerful resource in the change process. With this power comes the issue of confidentiality and the potential problem of secrecy. Most important for the systemically oriented therapist to understand and avoid is the easy trap of collusion, or re-creating the same relational dynamics that brought the clients into therapy in the first place.

The following example illustrates how collusion can develop. An anxious client calls you to make an appointment for therapy in order to talk about her husband. You schedule the appointment with her alone and listen to her story, which includes news that she's been having an affair with a family friend for the past 5 months. She thinks her lover is going to end the relationship and she's very uncertain as to what to do next. "Part of me wants to make my marriage work, of course, but my husband can't know about the affair, so I want you to promise not to tell him when I bring him in for some marital counseling." If the therapist quickly reassures the client that information is confidential and then begins therapy without addressing the impact of the secret, collusion has occurred. More important, the therapist has given over an important domain of powerful information to the client, without participating in defining how the secret might affect clinical work. Like resistance, collusion will occur. The therapist, however, must determine and actively participate in the control of pertinent information. Without this, the therapist is working with one arm tied behind his or her back.

Some therapists manage this dilemma by not allowing any confidential information to be disclosed—all sessions are with all family members and any phone contact will be disclosed in the next therapy session. Some therapists respect the confidential nature of information and determine that sometimes they will hold the confidence providing it doesn't interfere with therapeutic work. Some family therapy theories would say that secrets are mostly powerful in a negative way. Bowenian theory might see secrets as helping to create pathology in a subsequent generation; therefore, disclosing any secret would be therapeutic. Other theories, such as emotionally focused therapy, might be less interested in how truth was managed in the past and wholly interested in the honest sharing of emotional and behavioral information within the therapy session.

Again, one's clarity of theoretical focus as well as what is needed to maintain the therapeutic alliance must be evaluated in order to manage family secrets constructively.

HOW AGENCIES CONTRIBUTE TO BEING STUCK

Although family therapy has gained visibility and respect over the past several decades, it's a relatively new kid on the block within the mental health world. Agencies and institutions have developed to serve the needs of individuals, but they need to adapt to accommodate the different epistemology of systems thinking. For example, does the agency allow a therapist to keep a "family file" or does each family member need to be assessed individually—that is, given a diagnosis or mental status exam? Does the agency have senior supervisors familiar with the theory and practice of family therapy? Practically, do the rooms of the agency provide enough space or evening and weekend office hours to serve the needs of the family? Without considering these concerns, an agency's organization might interfere with effective treatment of the whole family.

Beginning family therapists need to be aware of the agency's level of commitment to systems-oriented therapy before beginning their work. In this way, expectations and change can be facilitated positively. As in doing good therapy, know who is supportive of family therapy, explore their position within the agency as a whole, and enter the system respectful of its power base. When significant change is needed, be willing to serve as a helpful partner in that change, perhaps by offering to review and edit intake forms. Offer your own perspective about the cases you observe or nondefensively ask for feedback regarding alternative theoretical positions, after explaining how you're dealing with a case. Find family therapy supports outside the agency if you're working as a Lone Ranger (even he had Tonto).

Interestingly, the most resistant cases appear when all systems involved—client, therapist, and agency—get stuck together. This is called isomorphism, a reference to the creation of similar relational structures across several systems. Client, therapist, and supervisory systems exist from the beginning of therapy. Since systems tend to re-create themselves at several levels, and beginning therapists are accountable across several systems, at times problems at one system level can be observed at another level. For example, a wife presented the problem of feeling powerless to change her husband; the therapist tried several interventions to help her respond differently to her husband, but she continued to do things in the same style; the supervisor directed the therapist to use another modality of therapy with this woman, but the therapist wanted to stay with the current agenda for a few more sessions. What we see at these three system levels is isomorphism, or similar interactional styles developing across systems. Isomorphism sometimes can be positive, but it also can signal areas of stuckness in the therapeutic relationship. Consider the case of Carl, a family therapist, and his client Bob. Carl has some difficulties in his work setting, which in turn have a direct effect on Bob's process of recovery.

Bob, a 32-year-old Caucasian male, reluctantly admits himself to an inpatient substance abuse program. His wife has been threatening to divorce him, and his employer indicates that Bob's work performance has suffered due to his alcohol-related absences. Bob feels that he drinks recreationally and can handle his problems. He does agree that he shouldn't drink so much during the week and thinks he can control it. He has even "quit completely several times, for 2 or 3 months." He thinks his wife should be more understanding of the stress that he's under because of his work and concentrate on her own problems. His fear of losing his job and his wife motivates him enough to enter a treatment program. His presentation is sarcastic, and he's resentful that he has to be there. He says that he'll stay for a while because he promised his wife. When asked about his goals he says, "I'm still trying to figure out why I'm here and who is in charge."

Bob's therapist is Carl, a 40-year-old Caucasian marriage and family therapist and a recovering alcoholic who has been working in the substance abuse field for the past 7 years. He has been sober for 12 years. Carl is a very committed professional who believes in combining the 12-step program with psychotherapy in order to help clients achieve sobriety. He works long hours and gets a great deal of satisfaction from his job. He feels that he has a realistic picture of what can be accomplished in treatment given "the time limits and nature of the disease of alcoholism."

Carl has worked with many clients like Bob who present an initial high degree of resistance to treatment and "denial as to the extent of their problem." Carl expects that Bob's hostility will begin to dissipate once he gets involved in some group meetings and begins to accept his problems.

In their first meeting, some of Bob's anger is directed at Carl. Bob insists that Carl can't really understand him and that he is only interested in keeping him in the hospital so that he can keep his job. Carl's response is to maintain his distance from Bob's anger and ask Bob further questions about his feelings about being in treatment. This helps to stop the attacks, but Bob continues to be fairly hostile throughout the session. In their second session Bob talks about his initial group meeting. He begins with sarcastic comments about some of the members and talks about why he doesn't think he belongs there. Further questions by the therapist help to identify some of Bob's feelings of identification with two of the group members who feel ambivalent about the treatment process. Carl's questions throughout the remainder of the session help Bob to disclose some of his fears about treatment. Carl leaves the second session feeling as though he has begun to develop a therapeutic alliance with Bob and the treatment process has begun.

Bob's treatment progresses well during the first week. He has quickly begun to like and respect Carl and is making good use of the treatment process. Carl also feels good about Bob's progress and begins to cautiously self-disclose about his own battle with alcohol. Carl sees some of himself in Bob, so he finds it a bit easier to talk with him than with most of the patients.

Toward the end of Bob's first week in treatment Carl begins to have some difficulties with his supervisor and some of the facility's policies. There has been a growing amount of required paperwork. The hospital has become more restrictive about overtime and has developed policies to discourage it. Carl's supervisor feels that his work with the patients is good but that his documentation is not up to par and he must improve in this area. Carl feels that his supervisor is more concerned about protecting his job than providing quality care, and he and the supervisor have a heated argument over this issue.

In his next meeting with Bob, Carl is still upset about his meeting with his supervisor. Although he knows better, he begins to talk about some of his frustrations with the hospital and his job. This becomes the topic of discussion for most of the session. Bob is very interested in Carl's difficulties with his job and asks lots of questions. Toward the end of the session he indicates that he has had some of the same kinds of problems with his boss.

At his next group meeting, Bob announces that he's going to leave the treatment program. He says he has learned that the program "doesn't have its priorities straight" and he doesn't "belong there."

The key for a beginning therapist, or any therapist, is to recognize when an isomorphic process is occurring. Unchecked, isomorphisms can be detrimental to therapy. With recognition comes the ability to be a more effective agent of change for the client.

COUNTERTRANSFERENCE: HOW THERAPIST ISSUES INTERFERE

Sharon was a 25-year-old intern who had been working comfortably with latency and teenage youngsters at a family service agency. One afternoon, Sharon met with the mother of a 7-year-old female client. The woman was very critical of the child and had unrealistic expectations of her daughter. Sharon thought the mother was expecting the girl to be "perfect," and she felt protective of the child. She identified with the little girl and noticed that the mother's criticism and demands reminded her of her relationship with her mother. Recognizing this connection, Sharon was able to disengage from a power struggle with the mother and maintain her composure through the rest of the session. Later, she sought supervision and was able to get help in separating her reactions to the client's mother from those toward her own mother.

These processes, which regularly come into play in therapy, stem from what analytically oriented therapists term "transference" and "countertransference." Often ignored or relabeled in family therapy texts, they relate to a phenomenon that is often discussed in supervision. Family therapy, in its attempt to establish its own specialization separate from psychoanalytic roots, tends to be more technique-focused and less concerned about the therapeutic relationship. More recent writings in family therapy, such as narrative therapy, have asked important questions concerning the interpersonal context of therapy. Certainly, it is in the interpersonal arena that self and family are shaped.

In very simple terms, transference denotes the interpersonal material brought into the therapeutic relationship by the client, and countertransference denotes the interpersonal material brought into the therapeutic relationship by the therapist. Object relations theories understand these components as the essential working domain for therapy, since in transference the client offers a re-creation of the affective, behavioral, and cognitive issues that need to be reworked for positive growth to take place. Countertransference, too, must be internally monitored and interpersonally used for therapeutic progress to occur.

Whatever terms are used, part of the process of therapy (especially when it lasts for some time) involves the way feelings, behaviors, and cognitions from the past are played out in the current therapeutic setting. For example, a single mother comes in to therapy for treatment of her depression. After several weeks of work in which the therapist empathizes with her situation and encourages access to underused resources in her life, she becomes more quiet and occasionally says, "I know you're going to get mad at me, but ... " The client expects the therapist will react to her just as her own mother had—with criticism and disappointment at her lack of progress.

Feelings, thoughts, and behaviors also emerge from the therapist's past. Almost weekly, in supervising practicum students, we hear the words "I thought I had my father (or mother, or boyfriend, or ex) in the room with me during part of the session."

In managing transference and countertransference, it is important first to normalize personal reactions during therapy. Note that these phenomena will probably occur more often when doing individual therapy than when doing couple or family work, because in the latter, several persons can serve the purpose of projective identification, that is, expecting someone other than the therapist to act as someone significant from one's own background.

Second, several common, though varied, themes can be understood in this process, including helplessness, control, and sexuality. Most often these themes develop when there's some form of anxiety in the system—a normal reaction to any change process. Some clients present with a "help me" cry that seems stronger than "I need help"; these clients readily stay in a victim stance even when they're no longer being victimized. A common therapist reaction is to feel overwhelmed by the client. For example, one intern remarked, "I found myself making phone calls to this family and worrying about them before I went to sleep at night. They were all consuming."

We do have many clients in this work who are in great pain and need, and compassionate reactions must be a part of what we do. However, good therapy requires that a working relationship be established in which each member of the system shares in therapy's progress. Without this working alliance, a client might remain stuck as a victim and the therapist will be "burned out" by the client system. Each client's responsibility for the therapy will need to be reviewed and clarified if the helplessness theme continues.

A control issue is present when one member of the system demands or dictates to everyone where the therapy should or should not go. If the client initiates control, then commonly the therapist feels criticized or incompetent. Young therapists, in particular, often look for approval from their clients as a way to feel adequate. Working with a demanding and critical client can distract the therapist from the job of facilitating change within the entire system. Further, the therapist might be pulled to react as other family members have acted, perhaps passively. It's important for the therapist to know his or her limits and actively acknowledge them. Beginning therapists need to feel comfortable about stating they are just that—beginning. As long as the therapist is backed up by solid, supportive supervision, this is fairly easy to do.

Therapists can inadvertently contribute to this controlling theme. Feeling internal pressure to be "in charge" may undermine a therapist's ability to share with clients the responsibility for doing the work necessary for change. Also, paradoxically, controlling persons need to be "reframed" as the most vulnerable or out of control. Controlling persons often are highly needy individuals and must be treated with care. If a therapist discovers that this is his or her style, it would be critical to examine the roots of this attitude in order to facilitate a more therapeutic alignment with the family.

The third theme is sexuality. Particularly in opposite-gender therapeutic relationships, romantic or erotic messages may be verbally or nonverbally introduced into the session. Therapists might be attracted or scared by this. Many interns have disclosed that they have sexual dreams about their clients. Several important aspects of the sexuality theme can be noted. First, gender issues are a part of all human relationships; this can't be avoided. Further, some people sexualize these gender factors, especially when they have been abused or are needy in this area. Finally, the emotional legacy from one's family of origin influences how comfortably or uncomfortably this domain will be addressed within the therapeutic relationship.

As a general rule, seeking therapy or peer consultation must be a part of professional development no matter how much experience one has. Therapy will be "loaded" if one's family of origin issues touch the clients with whom one works. All therapists have an Achilles' heel in their work, but using vulnerable parts of ourselves in our work can enhance and enrich the therapy greatly.

Finally, recognizing what type of work one does well, given certain family of origin experiences, provides a solid focus for one's energies. Learning about oneself is a lifelong journey, and this profession provides a wonderful context for continuing down this path.

DEALING WITH CLIENTS WE DISLIKE

Sooner or later you will have a client that you dislike. This is a problem that all therapists encounter. Unfortunately, disliking a client can undermine therapy. For example, it may lead a therapist to favor one member of a couple or family more than another, leading clients to feel that the therapist is not balanced in terms of advocating for all parties equally. Therapists may dislike a client for a number of different reasons, which may require them to respond with different strategies (Williams & Day, 2007).

One possible reason that a therapist may dislike a client is due to countertransference issues. Does the client remind you of someone in your life with whom you had a difficult relationship (e.g., parent, sibling, significant other)? Or, has the client harmed someone (e.g., child abuse, domestic violence, infidelity), reminding you of a similar experience? Does the client belong to a group of people (race/ethnicity, sexual orientation, religion, etc.) toward whom you have negative feelings? Answering yes to these questions might point to countertransference issues, which should be addressed through supervision and perhaps personal therapy. In more extreme cases, a referral to another therapist might be in the client's best interest.

In many cases, a negative response to a client may be diagnostic, providing important assessment information. For example, if you feel irritated by a client who is constantly blaming others, then it may help to recognize that the client has a poor external locus of control. A client who is irritable and critical may be suffering from depression. In other situations, you may find that your relational dynamic with the client you dislike parallels the process or dynamics that others within the family or couple have with the client. Recognizing the underlying clinical issue or parallel process often gives you greater objectivity about the client, reducing a sense of dislike for the client.

Our perception of a client can also be shaped by how others see the individual. Other people's negative feelings about a client could negatively affect our view of the client, particularly if we hear these negative views prior to meeting the individual. Conversely, it may be helpful to identify what others who like the client value about the individual. This may open us up to seeing some of the individual's positives that we have overlooked.

The therapist's initial response to a client may be one of dislike or anxiety, but looking further at the client's underlying concerns may help change the therapist's perspective. An angry or blaming person may be experiencing hurt, rejection, or fear underneath. Individuals with fragile self-esteem may have developed ways of compensating for this (e.g., being narcissistic) that make them difficult to like. Clients may initially present with a protective shield in order to help manage their fears and anxieties about the therapeutic process. One such client was a 40-year-old man who came to his initial session proclaiming that the therapist had three visits to make things better or he would stop coming to therapy. The client's statement was his way of maintaining control and managing his anxiety. Initially, it was important to join with the client, to help him feel safe and reassure him that he was in control of making changes. Once this occurred, he was able to be more vulnerable in disclosing his concerns. His timetable became less of an issue once he felt understood by the therapist and felt that he could impact what happened in the therapy.

A variety of other approaches can also help you deal with clients that you dislike. Actively seeking out client strengths can help counter negative feelings for a client. In some cases, a negative attribute (stubbornness) can be framed in a more positive light (perseverance). Therapists sometimes struggle liking individuals who have harmed others (e.g., child abuse, domestic violence). In these situations, it may be helpful to separate the person from the problem. One phrase that illustrates this philosophy is "God hates the sin, but loves the sinner." Separating the person from the problem allows one to be compassionate for the individual, yet avoid minimizing the destructiveness of the behavior. You may also need to develop greater empathy for the client by trying to learn more about his or her life. Often you will learn about challenges, life experiences, or other contextual factors that influence the client's behavior. Understanding the multigenerational context of an individual may be especially helpful in developing a greater (and more empathic) understanding of the client. Supervision is also recommended if you struggle with liking a client. Your supervisor may be able to offer a different perspective on the client. In many cases, clients that therapists dislike are also difficult to treat. Your supervisor may be able to offer some guidance on how to approach a difficult case, which might reduce your frustration with the client.

CONCLUSION: A FINAL REMINDER

Finding oneself stuck, for whatever reason, in the midst of the therapeutic process is ubiquitous in the early stages of one's work. Keep in mind that every point of "stuckness" provides a chance to increase competence and confidence. This chapter has identified some of the most common places therapists encounter challenges, and we've talked about ways to become "unstuck." Heightening awareness of the therapeutic process and developing specific skills, and knowing what steps to take when we meet obstacles, are the essential parts of our work.

CHAPTER 11

Termination

An important part of therapy is termination, even though it does not receive much attention in the literature; this is comparable to learning how to drive but never learning how to properly park the car and turn off the engine. A successful termination to therapy can be important for several reasons.

Terminations can be an effective way of empowering both the clients and the therapist. A successful termination should consolidate or reinforce the therapeutic gains of the client. For those who need to be referred or transferred, a successful termination can increase the likelihood that they will have a productive experience with a new therapist. For you as the therapist, a successful termination can help you understand how you were most helpful to the client, thereby building your confidence.

Terminations can also be important because they bring closure to the therapist–client relationship, an especially vital consideration in cases where the client and therapist have developed a strong connection over time. If properly handled, terminations can help clients and therapists deal with losses associated with ending the therapeutic relationship.

This chapter will discuss three types of terminations: client terminations, therapist terminations, and mutual terminations. Client terminations occur when the client unilaterally decides that therapy is over, whereas therapist terminations happen when the therapist unilaterally decides therapy should be discontinued. Mutual terminations occur when both the client and therapist agree on the termination, which typically occurs when both feel that client goals have been achieved.

Although these terminations will be discussed as three distinct phenomena, it is perhaps more accurate to view them on a continuum. Client and therapist terminations could be considered the two ends of the continuum, with mutual terminations representing the midpoint. Therefore, the therapeutic considerations outlined under each type may also partially apply to others, depending upon the situation.

MUTUAL TERMINATIONS

Most therapists strive for mutual terminations, where both you and your client are in agreement that the issues have been properly resolved and that continuing therapy is no longer necessary. In rare cases, both you and your client may agree that therapy should no longer be continued, but not necessarily because the issues are resolved. In one such example, both the therapist and client agreed that the client should discontinue therapy until she had finished a particularly difficult semester since most of her energy was devoted to finishing her studies. The client resumed therapy after completing her semester and had more energy to devote to her personal growth at that time.

When to Terminate

Although clients will sometimes bring up the topic of termination, it is often the therapist who must initiate a discussion about ending therapy. Therefore, it is important that you recognize when it is time to begin termination.

Mutual terminations generally result from having successfully achieved the goals for therapy. It will be easier to recognize when to conclude therapy if these goals have been clearly defined. If not, you may need to rely on other indicators. If your clients have difficulty finding issues to discuss in therapy, this is often a sign that therapy is close to ending. Likewise, if you and your clients spend a lot of time in session in nontherapeutic talk or social chatter, termination should be considered.

One of the difficulties that can arise when considering termination with couples or families is that not all family members may feel equally ready for terminating therapy. Sometimes this is simply due to family members having different levels of confidence in their ability to handle problems as they arise without the therapist's guidance. Usually the most effective approach is to space out the sessions until all family members have developed the confidence to end therapy.

In other cases, family members may not be in agreement about terminating therapy because they have different expectations about what they want to achieve through therapy. In these cases, you are faced with the same dilemma as when clients enter therapy with different expectations. It is often possible for you to help the couple or family achieve some compromise. In one case, a couple had made significant changes in eliminating their high level of conflict. The husband reported being satisfied with the changes that had been made and expressed interest in discontinuing therapy. While the wife agreed that the relationship was much improved, particularly in terms of the original goal of reducing conflict, she also expressed a desire to continue in therapy to improve the couple's sexual intimacy. A compromise was reached wherein the couple contracted to work on improving their sexual intimacy but agreed to come to therapy every other week rather than weekly, as they had previously done.

Termination Goals

In terminating therapy, it's helpful to keep three goals in mind. The first is to help clients consolidate the gains they have made through therapy. Termination should reinforce the new skills, behaviors, or ways of thinking that the clients have learned.

The second goal of termination is to empower clients, giving them greater confidence in their ability to manage their issues on their own in the future. Another result of empowerment is that there will be a leveling of power between the therapist and the clients, reducing the clients' dependence on you and increasing their self-reliance.

The third goal is to be sensitive to loss issues associated with terminations. Many clients develop a close relationship with their therapist and feel a sense of loss about ending the relationship. This is most likely to occur when you have worked with an individual, although at times couples or even families may have this experience. The sense of loss may be particularly keen for an individual who has a limited social support network to compensate for the loss of the therapeutic relationship.

Like clients, you may also experience a sense of loss when terminating therapy with certain clients. Therapists sometimes develop a very strong connection with certain clients, triggering feelings of sadness that the relationship is ending. These feelings can be compounded by other losses you may be experiencing. For example, when they leave their training program by virtue of graduation, many beginning therapists report sadness about ending relationships not only with clients that they care about, but also with colleagues and friends. You need to be prepared to acknowledge and deal with these feelings as they arise.

Termination as Process

Terminations are more successful if they are conceptualized as a process rather than as events. When viewed from this perspective, termination is not confined to the final session but is a process that ideally begins earlier. In fact, one could argue that the goals for termination should be in the therapist's mind from the initial session. A therapist who is aware that a client has a very limited support network could anticipate that the client is likely to develop a strong dependence on him or her. This in turn will make termination a more acute loss for the client. In fact, clients who are overly dependent upon their therapist may manufacture problems to prolong the therapeutic relationship. Therefore, a therapist in this case would be wise to help the client develop a stronger support network during therapy. This will not only empower the client by giving him or her more resources, but will reduce the feelings of loss since the client will have others to turn to for emotional support.

Therapeutic Interventions in Termination

You can use several interventions to help achieve the goals for termination. One common intervention is to begin spacing out sessions. This strategy can give your clients time to consolidate the gains they have made, and it also begins to build clients' confidence that they are managing problems on their own, since they have less contact with you.

In helping clients consolidate what they have gained from therapy, a number of questions can be asked. You can request that clients articulate what has changed for them and what they believe accounts for the change, or you can put them in the expert role by highlighting how successful they have been in addressing the problem and asking them for advice on how to work with other clients who have a similar difficulty. This approach has the advantage of empowering your clients in addition to helping them consolidate therapeutic gains. When asking clients to indicate what has brought about the changes, it's important that you give them permission to acknowledge things that may have happened outside of therapy. Some clients have difficulty answering the question of what they are doing differently. One possible approach to this problem is to ask them what they could do to make things worse, which often gives them insights into what positive changes have occurred (Hoffman, 1981). In other cases, you may need to help highlight for your clients the changes they have made.

It's often helpful to clients to predict temporary relapses. Clients can be told that change is a matter of "two steps forward and one step back." This helps them be less threatened by temporary setbacks, which in turn provides greater confidence in their ability to manage problems on their own.

Clients respond very positively when you can share something special that they have taught you. This is an effective way to empower your clients, making them feel the relationship has been reciprocal. For example, one therapist told a couple how a particular metaphor that had emerged out of their work together had been helpful in his work with other clients. As with any intervention in therapy, the therapist must be sincere and not simply manufacture something.

Some therapists also like to give small gifts to clients to mark termination. The gifts should be of little monetary value so clients do not feel obligated to give a gift in return; rather, the gift should be rich in symbolic meaning. One therapist gave a couple an onion to symbolize the different layers they had explored and the emotions that therapy elicited. The onion provided a focal point for the therapist and couple to process the end of an important relationship. The gift could also be a reminder of an important therapeutic theme.

Special Issues in Termination

One special issue that can arise at termination is whether to accept gifts from clients. Some therapists believe they should not accept any gifts from clients under any circumstances. Others believe that it's permissible to accept gifts from clients provided they aren't expensive. The advantage of not accepting any gifts is that you are never placed in the position of having to decide if a gift is too expensive to accept. The disadvantage of refusing to accept a gift is that it may hurt the client's feelings, particularly if the gift was meant to be a symbolic gesture. Therapists who are willing to accept gifts must weigh the monetary and symbolic meaning of the gift. This makes the judgment more difficult, but gives you more options in how to respond. Each therapist must make a personal choice on which philosophy he or she will adopt regarding gifts from clients.

Another issue that can arise at termination is that clients may want to continue to have a relationship with you outside of therapy. We recommend that you avoid this situation. It is not uncommon for clients to return to therapy because of new problems that arise. If you begin a relationship with your clients after termination and they need to resume therapy, it puts you in the uncomfortable position of having a dual relationship with them. Therefore, a major reason to avoid a relationship after termination is to preserve your clients' right to return to therapy if needed.

Avoiding relationships outside of therapy not only protects the clients, but it can also protect you. If problems arise in the relationship outside of therapy for any reason, you are vulnerable to having your professional behavior questioned. A therapist who gets romantically involved with a client after terminating therapy could be accused of taking advantage of the client if the relationship sours.

Finally, another issue that therapists sometimes face is clients who do not wish to terminate, but who would like to continue therapy on a less frequent basis. Some therapists see this request as a sign that the client is too dependent upon the therapist. Other therapists believe that this arrangement is completely appropriate and desirable for some clients. Some therapists advocate booster sessions to help maintain treatment gains.

When clients ask to continue therapy, you should carefully evaluate the motivation behind the request. The request may indeed signal excessive dependence upon you, particularly if your clients ask to see you on a frequent basis (more than once or twice a month). These clients typically have few people other than their therapist with whom they feel closely connected. You may then want to help your clients develop their support network to reduce their dependence on you.

However, the request to continue therapy doesn't always signal dependency issues. Some clients want to see their therapist periodically to help keep their family relationships healthy. For these clients, therapy is like going to the dentist for a 6-month preventative checkup. Other clients genuinely want to continue to grow, and they see therapy as a way to facilitate that growth. Therapy assumes more of a coaching or mentoring role, rather than a crisis or problem-solving role. Therefore, a therapist could feel comfortable seeing these clients periodically as a preventative measure or to facilitate the clients' desire for continued growth. For example, one of us (L. W.) continued to see a couple once every 3 months to facilitate the couple's continued growth and enrichment of their relationship.

THERAPIST TERMINATIONS

There will be times when a therapist may unilaterally decide therapy should be discontinued. As with client terminations, there can be a variety of reasons leading to a therapist termination. A common reason is that you are moving or terminating employment with an agency. In some instances, a therapist may wish to end therapy with particular clients due to specific issues in the case. The therapist may feel unqualified to deal with the issues, or feel that personal issues interfere with the case.

You might also suggest terminating therapy if agreement cannot be reached on the therapeutic contract or you strongly suspect the clients are not ready for change. However, you should work closely with these clients to make termination of therapy as much of a mutual decision as possible. In one case, for example, a therapist felt it was necessary to address the husband's severe mistrust of his wife as part of the couple's dynamics. However, the husband never agreed with the therapist's assessment that this was an important issue to address, creating an impasse in therapy. The therapist discussed with the couple how the lack of agreement on this key issue probably precluded a successful outcome to therapy. The couple agreed, resulting in a mutual decision to terminate therapy and a referral to another therapist for a second opinion.

When terminating therapy, you should give your clients as much notice as possible. Having therapy abruptly terminated is stressful for clients, particularly for those who have abandonment issues. Giving advance notice will give your clients time to prepare emotionally for the termination. Clients that you anticipate may particularly struggle with terminations may be informed even as early as 2–3 months in advance, if possible. This permits you to solicit and process your clients' fears regarding changing therapists. Advance notice of termination may also motivate your clients to work harder in therapy to avoid having to change therapists.

If the clients need to continue in therapy, then it is important that the therapist make a proper transfer or referral. When making an outside referral, ideally you will be able to provide your clients with at least three referrals so they have some choices. This increases the likelihood of the clients finding a suitable therapist. In other cases, clients can be transferred to another therapist within the same agency or practice.

Effectively transferring a case requires attending to the needs of the clients, departing therapist, and incoming therapist (Williams & Winter, 2009). Clients have multiple needs or concerns with regard to being transferred. For example, they need assurance that there will be continuity of care after you leave. If feasible, it is ideal if the new therapist can join you for at least one session prior to termination so that he or she can be introduced to the clients. You may even elect to do some type of intervention to mark the transition. For example, the incoming therapist may initially take an observing role during the transfer session but deliver a summarizing message at the end of the session to mark his or her assuming responsibility from that point forward. If a break in therapy is required because the new therapist is not immediately available, then your clients should be told when he or she will be available and whom to contact in the event an emergency should arise before then.

Clients may have several reservations about starting over with another therapist. Many, for example, may not want to tell their story over again. Even if you talk to the new therapist about the case, he or she will inevitably need to cover some history that was discussed in the previous therapy. Your clients' concerns about retelling their story can be validated, yet at the same time you can suggest that a fresh perspective may be gained by sharing some of the story again with a new person. Clients may also worry about whether they will like their new therapist. If you have had input on whom the new therapist will be, you can assure your clients that the incoming therapist has been selected with their needs in mind. It is also possible that your clients are concerned about whether the new therapist will like them. Offering reassurances that the new therapist will enjoy working with them can alleviate these fears, particularly if you can note the ways in which you have enjoyed working with the clients.

As with other terminations, it is important for you to review the progress your clients have made to date in meeting their goals. The transfer can be framed as closing one chapter and beginning a new one with the new person. As mentioned earlier, clients may experience a sense of loss over ending therapy. This will be particularly true for individuals who have a strong attachment to or dependence upon you. Some clients may also have anger about being transferred, which may or may not be expressed overtly. In some cases, this anger may be directed primarily at the new therapist. It is important that you or the new therapist not respond defensively to this anger or disappointment should it occur. Indeed, validating the feelings of loss and anger over a transfer may help the new therapist solidify the therapeutic relationship.

As the departing therapist, you also have important needs that should be considered in the process. As in other terminations, you may experience a sense of loss over therapy ending. A formal transfer or termination session can help bring proper closure for both you and the clients alike. You may also worry about the future welfare of your clients. In some cases, therapists may experience guilt because they worry that their clients' needs will not be met as a result of therapy ending. These feelings may be particularly strong if the therapist is unable to hand their clients over to another therapist that he or she knows or has confidence in.

The needs of the therapist receiving the transfer should also not be overlooked. The new therapist hopes that you can pass on a good understanding of the case. Ideally, both of you will be able to discuss the case prior to your departure. The new therapist can also review your case notes or consult with your supervisor to learn more about the case. Therapists receiving transfer clients can also struggle with issues of credibility, especially if they are less experienced. Ideally, you will be able empower the incoming therapist by highlighting his or her strengths or capabilities. With time, he or she can earn the clients' trust and credibility. The new therapist also needs to be able to renegotiate the contract for therapy. The goals for therapy, which may have changed over time, should be reviewed. Other expectations for therapy may also need to be renegotiated (e.g., approach to therapy, who will be in therapy, time or frequency of appointments). Asking clients what they liked and disliked about therapy can give the new therapist insight into what expectations they may be bringing into therapy.

CLIENT TERMINATIONS

Unilateral terminations, whether initiated by the client or therapist, are usually frustrating for the party that was not consulted. What can make client terminations even more difficult is that they can occur without warning, and the client may never offer an explanation for terminating therapy. The client may simply not show up for therapy, or might cancel the appointment and never reschedule. Therapist reactions to client terminations include blaming the client ("They were unmotivated"), being relieved ("They were a difficult case"), acceptance ("This happens to all therapists, it is just part of doing therapy"), or blaming oneself ("I must have done something wrong").

When a client does not return to therapy, beginning therapists frequently worry that they have done something wrong. However, you should not automatically assume that a termination is a sign of failure on your part (Ogrodniczuk, Joyce, & Piper, 2005). This point was poignantly made for one of us (L. W.) during two internship cases. One couple who had suddenly dropped out of therapy came back unexpectedly after 5 months. When he expressed surprise at seeing them return, they explained how a number of events such as a job change and move had made it difficult to continue therapy. However, they expressed eagerness to continue with therapy because they had found their earlier work together helpful.

A second couple came in approximately 2 weeks later, and reported that another couple had strongly recommended him based on their experience with him. He was surprised by the strong recommendation because the couple that had made the referral had dropped out of therapy unexpectedly.

Clients can terminate therapy for a variety of reasons (Renk & Dinger, 2002). For some clients, the problem may simply be resolved and they no longer see the need to continue therapy. As in the preceding example, you may get referrals from these clients even though they terminated somewhat unexpectedly.

Other clients simply may lose momentum in coming to therapy. They may cancel an appointment (due to illness) or promise to call later to reschedule (after returning from vacation or a business trip). For these individuals, therapy may have helped to partially resolve the problem. The clients may have obtained enough relief that they no longer feel compelled to reinitiate or continue with therapy.

Some clients may discontinue therapy because of external constraints. Financial hardships may keep some from returning. One man informed his therapist he could no longer afford the gas it took to come to therapy. Transportation difficulties, moving, changing jobs, or illness may be other reasons that clients discontinue therapy unexpectedly. A single mother who brought three young children to the first session did not return for a second session. When a follow-up phone call was made, she said getting to the agency by bus with three young children was stressful, and that she had found an agency that provided home-based services as an alternative.

Some clients will not return because they are dissatisfied with therapy. They may feel the therapist doesn't understand them or that change is not happening quickly enough. The dissatisfaction may be rooted in unrealistic expectations of what therapy is, or it may be because the therapist has been ineffective or has damaged the therapeutic relationship.

You should ideally follow up with clients who terminate without an explanation. Your next step will depend on the reason the clients terminated therapy. You might be able to negotiate a lower fee for clients who terminate for financial reasons. If you have harmed the therapeutic relationship, you can attempt to fix the relationship, or at a minimum provide referrals for your clients. In some cases, you might want to invite your clients in for a termination session to bring a proper closure to therapy.

CONCLUSION

Terminations can be a difficult time for clients and therapists alike, particularly if it is not mutually agreed upon by both parties. When the therapist must initiate termination, there is the potential for clients to feel abandoned or insecure about starting therapy with another therapist. Conversely, therapists may question whether they were effective in helping clients who appear to have prematurely left therapy. Even when terminating therapy is mutually agreed upon because goals for therapy have been successfully achieved, there can still be a sense of loss from ending the therapeutic relationship. An effective termination will deal with the losses and will also help clients consolidate the gains they have made and give them greater confidence about the future.

CHAPTER 12

Family Therapy in the Future

Pertinent Issues for Beginning Clinicians

Beginning family therapists exit graduate school and enter the mental health marketplace with a noble goal—to help clients alleviate their distress and suffering. But in the therapist's office of the 21st century, the challenge of doing therapy goes beyond the basics encountered during training. Clinical work in many settings means cooperating and sharing turf with other healthcare providers, giving increased attention to individual and DSM-IV-TR diagnoses, adhering to treatment guidelines provided by someone else, and complying with utilization reviews. More than ever, family therapists may find themselves playing double advocate roles: searching out creative options for clients whose healthcare plans limit modality and length of treatment, and helping the profession prove its legitimacy, thereby ensuring that family therapy is one treatment option.

As the second edition of this book goes to press, the United States is on the cusp of major healthcare reform, and mental health services will be one area where change occurs. In addition, many countries worldwide are struggling with how to pay for healthcare services. As countries struggle with economic reforms, leaders note the stresses that families face. In the global economy, government leaders look for ways to support families and children, including creating mental health services that support families. Whatever form the new systems take, family therapists can be certain the effects will be felt by themselves and their clients.

In the United States, there is tremendous variability by region in the availability of mental health services. We are hopeful that legislation supporting parity for mental and physical health means that more clients can receive treatment. Parity suggests that a client should have the same coverage (payment) for mental conditions that he or she has for physical conditions (Glied & Frank, 2008). Historically, many payers will not cover clients' mental health services even when they pay for physical care. Even if some mental health payment is offered, most insurance plans impose special limits on the amount of mental health care they will pay for.

Parity arguments usually center around cost sharing and "medical necessity." Even with private insurance, mental health clients are likely to pay a higher percentage for their mental health care than for physical care. "Medical necessity" generally refers to care that is accepted medical practice or meets community standards of care. Thus, payers do not want to pay for communication problems but are willing to pay for treatment of DSM diagnoses like anxiety, ADHD, depression, bipolar disorder, and schizophrenia.

In this chapter, we leave you with a glimpse of the present and future "business" of family therapy, the implications (pro and con) for your work with clients, and some pointers that will help you navigate the unpredictable waters of healthcare reform. In addition, we talk about trends in mental health services that will influence your work. Finally, we end the book with a discussion of the impact of your work as a therapist on you personally.

HEALTHCARE REFORM:
IMPLICATIONS FOR YOU AND YOUR CLIENTS

Healthcare reform may be both good news and bad news for consumers and providers of mental health services, and family therapists should be aware of both sides of the story. The good news is that a significant number of Americans who were previously uninsured will have access to care. Increasing access to care for these groups is a goal that resonates with the values of family therapists. The bad news is that there could be more pressure to identify a single client and provide treatments that are based on individual symptoms.

At the same time, clients and therapists may be caught in the ongoing battle to balance cost-effectiveness with quality care. The potential here is for postponed treatment, bureaucratic obstacles that lead clients to give up, and severely limited choices regarding who the clients can see. In addition, numerous chronic problems and certain acute ones may not qualify for treatment. Similarly, time-limited therapy may be the rule, despite the fact that resolution of some problems requires long-term treatment. Finally, in an environment where cost-effectiveness is so crucial, there may be an overreliance on drugs. The ease with which certain popular drugs are prescribed, and the use of these as diagnostic tools, may prevent clients from pursuing other types of treatment.

While these issues are significant for adult clients and their therapists, they are even more challenging for therapists who treat children and adolescents. Evidence for the critical importance of excellent care for children and adolescents comes from a national study examining the frequency of mental health problems (Kessler et al., 2005). In general, the research suggests that half of all mental health disorders start by age 14 and three-fourths start by age 24. In fact, the mean age for anxiety disorders and impulse disorders to start is 11 years old.

In spite of numerous efforts, children and adolescents are still frequently treated individually and the impact of their families is often overlooked. Nowhere is this more apparent than in the rush to provide psychotropic medications for children and adolescents as the first-line treatments. While we recognize the tremendous difference that medications have made, such as stimulants to treat ADHD, we hope that you will continue to advocate for the critical importance of family-based treatments for developing children and adolescents.

Master's-level family therapists may have an advantage in the emerging healthcare market, as do master's-level nurse practitioners and certified physician assistants. Providing quality care for common problems in the least expensive way will be fundamental to the new healthcare organization. Family therapists are likely to practice on a team with clinical psychologists, psychiatrists, and primary care physicians in order to address the healthcare needs of a population. The closer the family therapist is to the primary care physician, the better a biopsychosocial approach to healthcare can be maintained.

When the primary care physician and family therapist work together around the care of a person and family, a greater efficiency of care will complement the quality of services. New models for integrating mental health providers with primary care physicians could flourish. At present, the strongest research supporting collaborative care has come from treating the depressed elderly (*www.integratedprimarycare.com, www.cfha.net*). In addition, government organizations and foundations have created models of care for clients with little or no private insurance. Most models of collaborative care share a problem-solving focus, are brief (5 to 7 sessions), and may or may not include psychotropic medications as part of the treatment. While the traditional private practice model that focuses on self-pay clients will continue, we anticipate that healthcare reform will financially support the new models of care based on principles of good collaboration between healthcare professionals.

The positive side of new payment models is that the therapist need not withhold treatment because the family cannot afford therapy. The negative side is that some treatments deemed necessary by the therapist may still not be covered, while others may be time-limited. Family therapists need to use authorized sessions creatively, perhaps using alternatives to the standard of the weekly 50-minute hour. Since new payment models may put the burden of cost containment partially on the provider, family therapists must have some knowledge of case management and practice economics. Family therapists must be trained to think about issues regarding treatment efficiency, effectiveness, cost, client satisfaction, utilization, and access.

Thus, they must be able to work as part of an interdisciplinary team, which might include a primary care physician, a dietitian, a nurse practitioner, a psychiatrist, and any other healthcare specialist deemed necessary for effective treatment. Embedded in working as part of an interdisciplinary team are issues of loss of autonomy, establishing parity or hierarchical relationships with other healthcare providers, and credibility regarding the services provided by family therapy (compared to the more clearly measured outcomes of biological sciences and medical model treatments). Family therapists must understand how other specialists think about problems, for example, the psychiatrist's focus on individual physical symptoms or the family physician's focus on pragmatic, efficient treatment (Patterson et al., 2006; Patterson & Magulac, 1994). The ability to actively consult with and understand other professionals while communicating the role of family therapy is essential.

As part of healthcare reform, a specific diagnosis and treatment plan will be important. Because of utilization management, evidence-based outcomes research, and other macro-accountability methods, a clear articulation of the problem, possible treatments, chosen treatment, and expected outcomes is critical. In other words, family therapists need to convey appropriate information to payers and must be aware of specific criteria. For example, obtaining treatment authorization often includes the following: documenting a DSM-IV-TR diagnosis, level of impaired functioning, level of care needed, and prognosis. Proving medical necessity means addressing both diagnostic and functional criteria. While Axis I diagnoses indicate acuteness and medical need, the more chronic Axis II conditions may not be sufficient to obtain treatment authorization. Clinicians can focus on the acute manifestation of an Axis II disorder, which likely brought the client into therapy.

In addition to providing a DSM-IV-TR diagnosis, therapists may need to give evidence of clinical instability, which includes potential lethality to self or other, current medical status, and ability to perform basic self-care. In documenting authorizations, therapists will also address interpersonal relationships and a client's ability to maintain vocational and other activities—problems here might be classified as functional impairments.

While some diagnoses (e.g., phobias) have strict diagnostic criteria and convincing treatment outcome research, other issues frequently discussed in therapy are broader and may not be paid for. For example, most plans would not cover marital therapy to treat communication problems. However, a distressed spouse might tell his primary care physician that he is depressed and is not eating or sleeping because of a painful marriage. Part of the treatment for depression might be marital therapy. Whatever the identified problem and treatment goals, therapists need to use behavioral terms that reflect symptom reduction. Treatment modality also needs to be identified and rationalized using evidence-based guidelines.

In practical terms, family therapists need to identify and document the focus of treatment early, and use behavioral terms. Progress notes must be legible and up to date, and should demonstrate some measure of change noted from session to session. Further, therapists need to show reviewers that applicable treatment guidelines or current standards for treatment are being followed.

The relationship between continued therapy and client improvement is an important consideration. Group therapies that prove as effective as individual therapies may take precedence because they are cost effective. Using the Internet to provide client education and care could become more common. Since family therapists have been working with family groups and systems, they should already have the necessary skills to make this transition.

Finally, client satisfaction is important and can be measured using brief questionnaires. This should be an area where family therapists excel, since relationship skills have always been a basic ingredient of family therapy. Research suggests that patients' most frequent complaints and reasons for changing doctors include (1) the physician does not care, (2) the physician doesn't listen, and (3) the physician doesn't explain in a way that is understandable (Desmond, 1993). In like manner, therapists must communicate their caring and concern to their clients.

In the past, the family therapist's focus was on helping families function more effectively, usually by altering their interactions. Today, new family therapists must also think about cost-effectiveness, research effectiveness versus the practical efficacy of using a treatment in the "real world," criteria for treatment authorization, treatment guidelines, time-limited therapies, utilization reviews, and accountability. The approach may be interdisciplinary and biopsychosocial, and family therapists will become team members who share with other professionals a concern for the client's total health. By expanding beyond the boundaries of traditional family therapy training and gaining understanding of the forces shaping healthcare services, beginning family therapists can help themselves and their clients.

EMERGING TRENDS IN TREATMENT

While family therapy will always maintain its focus on family-based treatments and the biopsychosocial model, the field is also being shaped by broader influences and global changes. In this section, we identify some of the most important forces affecting family therapy. While these areas aren't always addressed in traditional curriculums, we believe that they will affect your future clinical work.

Evidence-Based Treatments (EBTs)

The previous section discusses payers' and the governments' interests in supporting proven, effective treatments. Physicians and therapists share these goals. Indeed, these goals have emerged into a movement in the United States. In every health discipline, professionals have supported the move toward evidence-based treatments (Mash & Hunsley, 2005; Hunsley, & Mash, 2005). EBTs refer to the integration of best research evidence with clinical expertise and client values when making treatment decisions (Sackett, Strauss, Richardson, Rosenberg, & Haynes, 2000). In Chapters 5 and 10, we discuss more about the process of finding the best treatment and give specific suggestions for the process. Evidence-based family therapy treatments include functional family therapy, multisystemic family therapy, structural family therapy, cognitive-behavioral couple therapy, emotionally focused therapy, and others. The movement toward EBTs suggests that reimbursement in the future will be tied to EBTs that have been proven effective for a specific problem. At present, problems are generally organized around DSM diagnoses.

If you have had little exposure to EBTs, opportunities exist for you to train yourself. In addition to learning the steps we mention in Chapter 10 under "Doing a Literature Search," training modules on the Internet can give you the basic skills to conduct a search on a client's problem or conduct a systematic review (*ebbp.org/training.html*). In addition, there are many EBT resources on the Web, including conference presentations, discussion groups, and expert discussions.

Family therapists may have concerns about the limits of EBTs (Patterson, Miller, Carnes, & Wilson, 2004; Williams et al., 2006). For example, therapists may feel that it takes too much time to conduct literature reviews. Another concern could be that the freedom to match the treatment to the individual client's circumstances is lost. Some therapists feel that EBTs are too reductionistic and don't capture the complexity of their clients' lives. Therapists are not alone in expressing concerns. One prominent physician states: "Numbers can only complement a physicians' personal experience ... as well as his knowledge of whether a 'best' therapy from a clinical trial fits a patient's particular needs and values" (Groopman, 2007, p. 6).

In spite of these concerns, we believe that the public and payers will increasingly demand EBTs. Thus, academic journals, professional organizations, and government agencies have created websites that provide information about EBTs. They have done the time-consuming research review for the therapists and succinctly summarized the findings into suggestions. Chapter 10 provides Web addresses for some of these summary sites. We recommend that you become familiar with this information and simultaneously maintain your focus on your clients' individual needs and circumstances.

Technology

In the previous section, we mentioned opportunities to teach yourself new skills by using resources on the Web. Technology, especially the Internet, has changed the way people obtain and use information. For family therapists and their clients the Web provides exciting new opportunities and some risks.

Many clients will have conducted their own search and will bring downloaded information about their problem to their initial therapy session. However, when searching for treatment options, they might have a difficult time distinguishing between safe, effective treatments and fraud. At times, our clients have mentioned the search they did using our name or our clinic's name so they would know about who we were before they had their first session. In addition, some treatment programs now exist exclusively online, and the only contact a client has with a therapist may be an occasional phone call.

The Internet is also a risk for our clients. Clients may ignore their family members because they spend each evening on blogs or chat rooms on the Web. They explore pornography and other high-risk websites. Clients may obtain wrong information about their problems or possible treatments on the Web.

In terms of opportunities, the Web offers a quick way to conduct a literature search on a specific topic. Besides the sites mentioned in Chapter 10, many Web resources are available for family therapists. For example, Google Scholar (*www.scholar.google.com*) is a free Web search engine that can search a wide variety of academic literature from many disciplines. Government-supported search engines like PubMed (*www.pubmed.gov*) and MedLine are free and offer access to a broad array of health literature. MedLine, the largest component of PubMed, indexes approximately 5,200 American journals and journals from over 80 other countries. A free tutorial is available on how to search PubMed (*www.nlm.nih.gov/bsd/disted/pubmedtutorial*). Simply searching some government websites of agencies such as the National Institute of Mental Health (*www.nimh.nih.gov*) or the Substance Abuse and Mental Health Services Administration (*www.samhsa.gov*) can also be helpful. Other article databases include Thomson ISI's Web of Science (*www.isiweb-ofknowledge.com*) and Wiley InterScience (*www3.interscience.wiley.com*). Many journals now publish their entire content online. Some of these resources require paid subscriptions, and some are free.

Besides using search engines, family therapists can attend lectures and receive online training. Besides the EBT training mentioned earlier, therapists can participate in live lectures on mental health problems via the Massachusetts General Hospital Psychiatry Academy (*www.mghcme.org*). Webcasts, audio and video podcasts, and expert online forums are available for free just by logging in. Training centers are also putting lectures online. For example, a family therapist can watch a lecture summarizing the unique role of marriage as a source of social support by going to the Pittsburgh Mind–Body Center (*pmbcii.psy.cmu.edu*).

Videoconferencing and other new communication tools are also available for therapists. Our colleagues are using Skype to provide supervision to family therapists in another country. One of the most exciting opportunities that new technologies provide is the chance to work with family therapists from around the world without having to travel to another country. Long-distance meetings and teaching can take place using videoconferencing.

Initiatives in medicine and mental health are exploring service delivery via the Internet and using cell phones, text messaging, and e-mail reminders for health promotion and prevention. Recent research has demonstrated that phone therapy had a much lower attrition rate than traditional therapy, and some clients prefer technology as a medium for therapy because of its convenience and anonymity (Mohr, Vella,

Hart, Heckman, & Simon, 2008). Family therapists who want to provide services to clients in rural areas are exploring using technology to conduct therapy sessions (Bischoff, Hollist, Smith, & Flack, 2004). Today, clients can find therapists who are willing to provide therapy via the Internet while some therapists see advanced technology as a way of expanding their practices.

However, family therapists should carefully consider the needs of their clients and their ability to provide uncompromised treatments through this medium. Given that the use of technology to provide treatment is evolving as quickly as the technology itself, state laws and regulations and ethical guidelines from professional organizations have not kept pace. International guidelines are nonexistent. Family therapists considering service delivery through the Internet or using other technology should keep abreast of the laws and regulations governing the practice of family therapy in both the state in which they are licensed and the state in which the client resides before entering into an agreement to provide treatment. Therapists should also carefully consider the limitations of using technology to deliver services and receive proper training prior to doing so.

Globalization

Globalization is a broad force influencing the future of family therapy and encouraging family therapists to become more competent in dealing with cultural diversity, economic disparities, and gender (Keeling & Piercy, 2007). The globalization of family therapy raises important issues. In different societies gender roles, views about alternative family forms, and the very definition of family often differ from American norms. For example, in many countries, when clients speak about family, they mean extended family, not the nuclear family. Furthermore, mental health services to treat disorders such as depression or ADHD have been nonexistent in many countries. In addition, many cultural practices "denote recurrent, locality-specific patterns of aberrant behavior ... that may or may not be linked to a particular DSM diagnostic category" (American Psychiatric Association, 2000, p. 898). In other words, the boundaries between cultural differences and mental disorders are not always clear. Increasing globalization means that the impact of culture on mental health services is becoming more important.

In general, family therapists outside the United States work in countries with developed economies. While there are AAMFT approved supervisors in many countries outside the United States, the majority live in Europe or Hong Kong. Professional organizations such as the International Family Therapy Association (*www.ifta-familytherapy.*

org), the European Family Therapy Association (*www.europeanfamilytherapy.eu*), and Asia's regional family-based professional organization, the Consortium of Institutes on Family in the Asian Region (*www.cifa-net.org*) are building their own communities of family therapy professionals. In addition, many regions have created their own family therapy journals such as the *Australia and New Zealand Journal of Family Therapy* (*www.anzjft.com*) or the *Journal of Family Therapy in the United Kingdom* (*www.aft.org.uk*).

In addition to developing awareness about gender, economic disparities, and cultural diversity in their home country, family therapists can expand to a global focus on families and their struggles. Becoming bilingual, using the Internet for teaching or supervision, cross-cultural teaching exchanges, and reading international literature about families and their struggles are all ways to become aware of global issues in family therapy.

There are numerous globalization efforts in family therapy. A family therapy training program in Hong Kong conducts live group supervision with a training program in Taiwan using video conferencing. Japanese colleagues translate a popular English-language family therapy text into Japanese. Colleagues from the International Family Therapy Association set up a voluntary program to send well-known therapists to clinics in countries with developing economies. Colleagues from Australia, Israel, and other countries publish their research in American journals. A university takes a group of family therapy students to a family therapy conference in Asia. Family therapy programs in the United States discuss the possibilities of creating joint training programs and offering joint degrees with family therapy clinics in Asia and Europe. Discussions about an international credential in family therapy occur between different stakeholders.

In the coming years, more countries will develop family therapy programs and create their own unique training programs and models. Family therapists of the future will have to tease out the universal characteristics of families and simultaneously identify regional differences. The impact of factors such as race, gender, culture, and class on family members' mental health will become even more complex. With the complexities of globalization come new intellectual challenges that can make a career as a family therapist even more interesting.

Genetics and Neuroscience

Some of the most exciting work for family therapists is taking place in disciplines that are traditionally associated with biology and other natural sciences. Research in genetics and neuroscience is providing new understanding of vexing problems. As with other mental health disciplines, family therapists have had to focus on observable signs and reported symptoms when they assess their clients' problems. This has meant that clients often do not receive treatment until problems are entrenched. Family therapists, like other health providers, focus on treatment, not prevention. Focusing on treatment alone can be frustrating because many family therapists have strong backgrounds in human development and recognize the powerful influence of family interaction. Is it possible for family therapists to intervene earlier, before problems and illnesses have caused disability and suffering?

Recent advances in neuroscience and genetics point to underlying biology as a powerful source of human suffering. However, the same research suggests that biology is not destiny. In fact, for many (but not all) mental illnesses, one's genetics are only part of the etiology. A Stanford professor of biology and neurology summarizes the age-old nature-versus-nurture argument by stating:

> Genes don't cause behaviors. Sometimes they influence them.... Genes influence behavior, environment influences behavior, and genes and environment interact ... the effects of a gene on an organism will usually vary with changes in the environment, and the effects of environment will vary with changes in the genetic makeup of the organism. (Sapolsky, 2005, p. 30)

Research in neuroscience has also begun to illuminate our understanding of mental disorders. For example, neuroscience research has pointed out that the brain is more malleable than scientists once thought. The plasticity of the brain and the fact that adult brains produce new neurons provide hope that changing the environment (such as creating a supportive, loving family environment) can influence family members' individual biology. Neuroscientists explore the influence of epigenetic factors, or the way the environment shapes gene expression. Some of the most interesting research about environment shaping biology, based on attachment theory, is called interpersonal neurobiology (Siegal, 1999, 2007; Schore, 2003a, 2003b, 2005). In a nutshell, this research suggests that a person's brain is wired for optimal development when the person receives love and nurture from a warm caretaker.

Other findings have suggested that early interventions might create important changes in human development. In animal studies, baby rats who were licked and groomed by their mothers (attachment behaviors) developed a stronger capacity to deal with stress as adults, and scientists demonstrated the neuropathways between attachment behaviors and stress regulation mechanisms in the brain (Insel & Quirion, 2005). Stated more simply, research indicates that "the neurons that fire together, wire together." Similar questions are being raised about the impact of families on children's emerging mental illnesses. For example, in research on bipolar disorder in children, "kindling theory" suggests that the first manic episode is more likely to be associated with major stressors than are later episodes, which implies that stress might change and reinforce pathways inside the central nervous system so that future episodes of mania will occur without an outside stimulus. In an attempt to prevent the child's brain from becoming increasingly sensitized and perhaps prevent the first manic episode, researchers are exploring whether family therapy can fortify a child against a genetic proclivity for bipolar disorder (Egan, 2008). Family therapists do not need to wait until research in genetics and neuroscience have explicitly explained the pathways of the interaction between biology and the environment. Instead, we can begin applying our current understanding of the family's impact on mental health by helping families create supportive, nurturing environments that minimize stress and negativity.

Much research in neuroscience and genetics is only emerging. However, as experts in family interaction and family development, family therapists will have exciting opportunities in the future. While some mental illnesses will remain intractable to psychosocial interventions, many other mental health problems can be ameliorated by creating healthy families, especially families that support and nurture their younger members. In this way, family therapists might become agents of prevention, not treatment. In a healthcare culture focused on cost-effective interventions, influencing children and adolescents in the context of their families makes sense—especially given the research suggesting that most mental health problems begin in childhood and adolescence. The chance to contribute to an understanding of how healthy family life contributes to healthy children is just one of the pluses of work as a family therapist.

THE PERSONAL AND PROFESSIONAL JOURNEY OF BEING A THERAPIST

One of the questions we ask our graduating master's-level students is where they see themselves in 5 years. Some respond with the hopes of a good job, some want to be in a doctoral program, and almost all want the opportunity to do therapy. The profession offers increasing possibilities in the public and private sectors. Jobs can be found doing clinical work, management, consulting, teaching, and working as an administrator.

Many therapists work in several settings. It is not unusual for a therapist to have a part-time job in an agency, school, or institution and have a part-time private practice. Teaching and consulting can be instrumental in providing challenging opportunities for professional colleagueship and exposure to current ideas in the field. Most therapists enjoy diversity in their work and have considerable freedom in establishing their workload and schedule. Exposure to clients with various life experiences and diverse backgrounds can add richness to the therapist's life.

At graduation, we also ask our students to think about their lives and how they would like to balance their personal and professional goals. We share some of the goals that we've had over the years and then we ask them what they wish they'd known when they started their training. Here are some issues they mention:

- "Graduate school in family therapy and clinical training took more of an emotional toll on my life than my general undergraduate education did."
- "Having a positive work environment is worth everything. I would be willing to take a lower-paying job to be in a setting where I feel valued and supported."
- "I realized that there is no point in doing this work if you don't love it because you'll be a therapist for a long time. In addition, I realize that being a therapist is a lifestyle, not just a job, because I'm working with humans whose needs don't stop when it is five o'clock."
- "Money and salary matters. When I started graduate school, I never thought about my future income. Now, as I face paying off student loans and supporting a family, I care a great deal about finding a job with a good salary."
- "Taking time for self-care and not making my clients my whole life is important. At first, I felt so overwhelmed by my clients' needs that I wouldn't take out time for myself. Eventually I realized that I had to have a break from my clients and my work if I was going to last in this profession."
- "Ultimately, my relationships with my own family and friends are the most important parts of my life. When I first started, I inadvertently ignored them because I was so focused on my clients' needs. As time passed, I realized that I wouldn't be happy if I didn't stay close to the people I love."

One of the unique aspects of being a therapist is the merging of one's personal and professional life. Therapists need to be aware of their personal boundaries and clear about how their personal lives can affect their work. In addition, most therapists readily acknowledge that their professional work influences the choices they make in their personal lives.

Doing therapy can also be emotionally draining and can at times cause the therapist to maintain some distance in personal relationships. Taking time to decompress and finding some self-soothing activities can help in this process. Therapists can get caught in the midst of their clients' struggles, and feel under attack if they are dissatisfied with their relationships or lives. Over time, therapists learn to recognize these experiences and find ways to respond to their clients and soothe themselves.

CONCLUSION

"I rarely hear my therapist colleagues complain that their lives lack meaning. Life as a therapist is a life of service to others" (Yalom, 2002, p. 256). The profession offers the therapist a consistent opportunity to learn from others, self-reflect, and be a part of life-changing experiences. Being a therapist gives you the opportunity to be in a creative environment. Doing therapy, each time, can feel like the unfolding of a new day. Most therapists rely heavily upon their intuition. Trusting one's own sense of things, as well as helping others make sense of their experiences, is a constant creative challenge. For many therapists, the interplay between a life of service and meaning plus the constant challenge of responding creatively to new problems makes any stresses of work as a therapist well worth the effort.

References

Achenbach, T. (2008). Assessment, diagnosis, nosology, and taxonomy of child and adolescent psychopathology. In M. Hersen & A. M. Gross (Eds.), *Handbook of clinical psychology: Vol. 2. Children and adolescents* (pp. 429–457). Hoboken, NJ: Wiley.

Ahrons, C. (1994). *The good divorce.* New York: HarperCollins.

Ahrons, C. R. (2007). Family ties after divorce: Long-term implications for children. *Family Process, 46,* 53–65.

Ahrons, C. R., & Rodgers, R. H. (1987). *Divorced families: A multidisciplinary view.* New York: Norton.

Alexander, J., Holtzworth-Munroe, A., & Jameson, P. (1994). The process and outcome of marital and family therapy: Research review and evaluation. In A. Bergin & A. Garfield (Eds.), *Handbook of psychotherapy and behavior change* (pp. 595–630). New York: Wiley.

Alexander, J. F., & Sexton, T. L. (2002). Functional family therapy: A model for treating high risk, acting out youth. In F. W. Kaslow (Ed.), *Comprehensive handbook of psychotherapy: Vol. 4. Integrative/eclectic* (pp. 111–132). New York: Wiley.

American Psychiatric Association. (2000). *Diagnostic and statistical manual of mental disorders* (4th ed., text rev.). Washington, DC: Author.

Amstadter, A. (2008). Emotion regulation and anxiety disorders. *Journal of Anxiety Disorders, 22*(2), 211–221.

Anderson, C. (2003). The diversity, strength, and challenges of single-parent households. In F. Walsh (Ed.), *Normal family processes* (3rd ed., pp. 121–152). New York: Guilford Press.

Anderson, C. M., & Stewart, S. (1983). *Mastering resistance: A practical guide to family therapy.* New York: Guilford Press.

Arkowitz, H., Westra, H. A., Miller, W. R., & Rollnick, R. (Eds.). (2008). *Motivational interviewing in the treatment of psychological problems.* New York: Guilford Press.

Baldwin, S. A., Wampold, B. E., & Imel, Z. E. (2007). Untangling the alliance-outcome correlation: Exploring the relative importance of therapist and patient variability in the alliance. *Journal of Consulting and Clinical Psychology, 75,* 842–852.

Baruchin, A. (2008, May 22). Nature, nurture and attention deficit. *New York Times.* Retrieved from *health.nytimes.com/ref/health/healthguide/esn-adhd-expert.html.*

Baucom, D. H., Hahlweg, K., & Kuschel, A. (2003). Are waiting-list control groups needed in future marital therapy outcome research? *Behavior Therapy, 34,* 179–188.

Beach, S. (2003). Affective disorders. *Journal of Marital and Family Therapy, 29,* 247–261.

Beach, S., & Gupta, M. (2005). Understanding and treating depression in couples. *Journal of Family Psychotherapy, 16*(3), 69–83.

Beach, S., & Gupta, M. (2006). Directive and nondirective spousal support: Differential effects? *Journal of Marital and Family Therapy 32*(4), 465–477.

Beach, S., & Jones, D. (2002). Marital and family therapy for depression in adults. *Handbook of depression* (pp. 422–440). New York: Guilford Press.

Beach, S., Wambold, M., Kaslow, N., Hegman, R., First, M., Underwood, L., et al. (2006). *Relational process and DSM-V.* Washington, DC: American Psychiatric Association.

Beidel, D. C., & Turner, S. M. (2007). *Shy children, phobic adults: Nature and treatment of social anxiety disorder* (2nd ed.). Washington, DC: American Psychological Association.

Belmaker, R. H., & Agam, G. (2008). Major depressive disorder. *New England Journal of Medicine, 358*(1), 55–68.

Berg, B., & Rosenblum, N. (1977). Fathers in family therapy: A survey of family therapists. *Journal of Marriage and Family Counseling, 3,* 85–91.

Berger, D., & Berger, L., (1991). *We heard the angels of madness.* New York: Morrow.

Bergin, A. (1991). Values and religious issues in psychotherapy and mental health. *American Psychologist, 46*(4), 394–403.

Bertalanffy, L. von. (1968). *General system theory.* New York: George Braziller.

Bischoff, R., Hollist, C., Smith, C., & Flack, P. (2004). Addressing the mental health needs of the rural underserved: Findings from a multiple case study of a behavioral telehealth project. *Contemporary Family Therapy, 26,* 179–198.

Bischoff, R. J., & Barton, M. (2002). The pathway toward clinical self confidence. *American Journal of Family Therapy, 30,* 231–242.

Blow, A. J., & Hartnett, K. (2005). Infidelity in committed relationships: II. A substantive review. *Journal of Marital and Family Therapy, 31,* 217–234.

Borum, R., & Reddy, M. (2001). Assessing violence risk in Tarasoff situations: A fact-based model of inquiry. *Behavioral Sciences and the Law, 19,* 375–385.

Bowen, M. (1978). *Family therapy in clinical practice.* New York: Jason Aronson.

Bray, J., & Kelly, J. (1998). *Stepfamilies: Love, marriage, and parenting in the first decade.* New York: Broadway Books.

Breen Ruddy, N., & McDaniel, S. H. (2008). Couple therapy and medical issues: Working with couples facing illness. In A. S. Gurman (Ed.), *Clinical handbook of couple therapy* (4th ed., pp. 618–640). New York: Guilford Press.

Brown, E. M. (1991). *Patterns of infidelity and their treatment.* New York: Brunner/Mazel.

Buck, J., & Jolles, I. (1966). *House-Tree-Person.* Los Angeles: Western Psychological Services.

Butler, M. H., Davis, S. D., & Seedall, R. B. (2008). Common pitfalls of beginning therapists utilizing enactments. *Journal of Marital and Family Therapy, 34,* 329–352.

Carey, B. (2006, December 22). Parenting as therapy for child's mental disorders. *New York Times.* Retrieved from *www.nytimes.com/2006/12/22/health/22KIDS.html.*

Carter, E. A., & McGoldrick, M. (1989). *The changing family life cycle* (3rd ed.). Boston: Allyn & Bacon.

Castle, D., Kulkarni, J., & Abel, K. M. (Eds.). (2006). *Mood and anxiety disorders in women.* New York: Cambridge University Press.

Cavedo, C., & Guerney, B. G. (1999). Relationship enhancement enrichment and problem-prevention programs: Therapy-derived, powerful, versatile. In R. Berger & M. T. Hannah (Eds.), *Preventive approaches in couples therapy* (pp. 73–105). Philadelphia: Brunner/Mazel.

Charny, I. W. (2006). Staying together or separating and divorcing: Helping couples process their choices. In C. A. Everett & R. E. Lee (Eds.), *When marriages fail: Systemic family therapy intervention and issues, a tribute to William C. Nichols* (pp. 21–36). New York: Haworth Press.

Clarkin, J. F., & Glick, I. (1992). *A manual for psychoeducational marital intervention of bipolar disorder.* New York: Cornell Medical Center.

Cohen, S. (2004). Social relationships and health. *American Psychologist, 59*(8), 676–684.

Connell, J. (1995, December 6). Bridging gap between faith and medicine. *San Diego Union–Tribune,* p. D-1.

Conners, C. K. (1997). *Conners' Rating Scale—Revised technical manual.* North Tonawanda, NY: MultiHealth Systems.

Cooper, A. (1998) Sexuality and the Internet: Surfing into the new millennium. *Cyber-psychology and Behavior, 1*(2), 181–187.

Cordova, J. V., & Gee, C. B. (2001). Couples therapy for depression: Using healthy relationships to treat depression. In S. R. H. Beach (Ed.), *Marital and family processes in depression: A scientific foundation for clinical practice* (pp. 185–204). Washington, DC: American Psychological Association.

Costello, J. E., Mustillo, S., Erkanli, A., Keeler, G., & Angold, A. (2003). Prevalence and development of psychiatric disorders in childhood and adolescence. *Archives of General Psychiatry, 60*(8), 837–844.

Crane, D., Newfield, N., & Armstrong, D. (1984). Predicting divorce at marital therapy intake: Wives' distress and the marital status inventory. *Journal of Marital and Family Therapy, 10*(3), 305–312.

Craske, M., & Zoellner, L. (1995). Anxiety disorders: The role of marital therapy. In N. S. Jacobson & A. S. Gurman (Eds.), *Clinical handbook of couple therapy* (pp. 394–410). New York: Guilford Press.

Dadds, M. (1995). *Families, children and the development of dysfunction.* Thousands Oaks, CA: Sage.

Davis, J. L., & Petretic-Jackson, P. A. (2000). The impact of child sexual abuse on adult interpersonal functioning: A review and synthesis of the empirical literature. *Aggression and Violent Behavior, 5,* 291–328.

Dell'Osso, B., Marazziti, D., Hollander, E., & Altamura, A. (2007). Traditional and newer impulse control disorders: A clinical update. *Clinical Neuropsychiatry: Journal of Treatment Evaluation, 4*(1), 30–38.

Denton, W., & Burwell, S. (2006). Systemic couple intervention for depression in women. *Journal of Systemic Therapies, 25*(3), 43–57.

Denton, W., Patterson, J., & Van Meir, E. (1997). Use of the DSM in marriage and family therapy programs: Current practices and attitudes. *Journal of Marital and Family Therapy, 23*(1), 81–86.

Desmond, J. (1993, October). *The physician–patient relationship.* Paper presented at the meeting title Managed Care: An Approach for the Physician, San Diego County Medical Society, San Diego, CA.

Dilsaver, S. C. (1990). The mental status examination. *American Family Physician, 41*(5), 1489–1497.

Doherty, W., & Simmons, D. (1996). Clinical practice of marriage and family therapists: A national survey. *Journal of Marital and Family Therapy, 22,* 9–25.

Drugs for Psychiatric Disorders. (2006). *Treatment Guidelines from the Medical Letter, 4*(46), 35–46.

Duncan, G. J., Dowsett, C. J., Claessens, A., Magnuson, K., Huston, A. C., Klebanov, P., et al. (2007). School readiness and later achievement. *Developmental Psychology, 43*(6), 1428–1446.

Dupree, W. J., White, M. B., Olsen, C. S., & Lafleur, C. T. (2007). Infidelity treatment patterns: A practice-based evidence approach. *American Journal of Family Therapy, 35,* 327–341.

Dutra, L., Stathopoulou, G., Basden, S. L., Leyro, T. M., Powers, M. B., & Otto, M. W. (2008). A meta-analytic review of psychosocial interventions for substance use disorders. *American Journal of Psychiatry, 165*(2), 179–187.

Duvall, E. (1955). *Family development.* New York: Lippincott.

Edwards, D. L., & Gil, E. (1986). *Breaking the cycle: Assessment and treatment of child abuse and neglect.* Los Angeles: Association for Advanced Training in the Behavioral Sciences.

Edwards, J., Johnson, D., & Booth, A. (1987). Coming apart: A prognostic instrument of marital breakup. *Journal of Applied Family and Child Studies, 36*(2), 168–170.

Edwards, M., & Steinglass, P. (1995). Family therapy treatment outcomes for alcoholism. *Journal of Marital and Family Therapy, 21*(4), 475–509.

Egan, J. (2008). The bipolar puzzle: What does it mean to be a manic depressive child? *New York Times*. Retrieved September 18, 2008, from *www. nytimes.com/2008/09/14/magazine/14bipolar-t.html*.

Engel, G. L. (1977). The need for a new medical model: A challenge for biomedicine. *Science, 196*, 535–544.

Essex, M., Kraemer, H., Armstrong, J., Boyce, W., Goldsmith, H., Klein, M., et al. (2006). Exploring risk factors for the emergence of children's mental health problems. *Archives of General Psychiatry, 63*(11), 1246–1256.

Estrada, A., & Pinsof, W. (1995). The effectiveness of family therapies for selected behavioral disorders of childhood. *Journal of Marital and Family Therapy, 4*, 403–440.

Etkin, A., & Wager, T. (2007, October). Functional neuroimaging of anxiety: A meta-analysis of emotional processing in PTSD, social anxiety disorder, and specific phobia. *American Journal of Psychiatry, 164*(10), 1476–1488.

Everett, C. A., & Volgy, S. S. (1991). Treating divorce in family-therapy practice. In A. S. Gurman & D. P. Kniskern (Eds.), *Handbook of family therapy, vol. 2* (pp. 508–524). New York: Brunner/Mazel.

Evidence-based behavioral-practice online training modules. (2007). Retrieved September 12, 2008, from *ebbp.org/training.html*.

Ewing, J. A. (1984). Detecting alcoholism: The CAGE questionnaire. *Journal of the American Medical Association, 252*, 1905–1907.

Fals-Stewart, W., Kashdan, T., O'Farrell, T., & Birchler, G. (2002). Behavioral couples therapy for drug abusing patients: Effects on partner violence. *Journal of Substance Abuse Treatment, 22*, 87–96.

Fals-Stewart, W., O'Farrell, T., Birchler, G. R., Cordova, J., & Kelley, M. L. (2005). Behavioral couples therapy for alcoholism and drug abuse: Where we've been, where we are, and where we're going. *Journal of Cognitive Therapy, 19*(2), 225–246.

Finkelhor, D., Hotaling, G., Lewis, I. A., & Smith, C. (1990). Sexual abuse in a national survey of adult men and women: Prevalence, characteristics and risk-factors. *Child Abuse, 14*, 19–28.

Fisch, R., Weakland, J. H., & Segal, L. (1985). *The tactics of change: Doing therapy briefly.* San Francisco: Jossey-Bass.

Fitchett, G. (1993). *Spiritual assessment in pastoral care: A guide to selected resources.* Decatur, GA: Journal of Pastoral Care Publications.

Franklin, K., & Herek, G. M. (2003). Violence toward homosexuals. In S. Plous (Ed.), *Understanding prejudice and discrimination* (pp. 384–401). New York: McGraw-Hill.

Ganong, L., Coleman, M., Fine, M., & Martin, P. (1999). Stepparents' affinity-seeking and affinity-maintaining strategies with stepchildren. *Journal of Family Issues, 20*, 299–327.

Garbarino, J., & Stott, F. (1989). *What children can tell us: Eliciting, interpreting, and evaluating information from children.* San Francisco: Jossey-Bass.

Glied, S., & Frank, R. (2008). Shuffling toward parity—bringing mental health care under the umbrella. *New England Journal of Medicine, 359*, 113–115.

Goldner, V. (1985). Feminism and family therapy. *Family Process, 24,* 31–47.

Gordon, K. C., Baucom D. H., & Snyder, D. K. (2004). An integrative intervention for promoting recovery from extramarital affairs. *Journal of Marital and Family Therapy, 30,* 213–232.

Gotlib, I., & Beach, S. (1995). A marital/family discord model of depression: Implications for therapeutic intervention. In N. S. Jacobson & A. S. Gurman (Eds.), *Clinical handbook of couple therapy* (pp. 411–436). New York: Guilford Press.

Gottman, J. M. (1994). *What predicts divorce?* Hillsdale, NJ: Erlbaum.

Gottman, J. M. (1999). *The marriage clinic.* New York: Norton.

Gottman, J. M, & Notarius, C. I. (2000). Decade review: Observing marital interaction. *Journal of Marriage and the Family, 62,* 927–947.

Gould, J. W., & Martindale, D. A. (2007). *The art and science of child custody evaluations.* New York: Guilford Press.

Grant, J. (2008). *Impulse control disorders: A clinician's guide to understanding and treating behavioral addictions.* New York: Norton.

Green, R.-J., & Mitchell, V. (2008). Gay and lesbian couples in therapy: Minority stress, relational ambiguity, and families of choice. In A. S. Gurman (Ed.), *Clinical handbook of couple therapy* (4th ed., pp. 662–680). New York: Guilford Press.

Greene, K., & Bogo, M. (2002). The different faces of intimate violence: Implications for assessment and treatment. *Journal of Marital and Family Therapy, 28,* 455–466.

Griffith, J. L., & Griffith, M. E. (1994). *The body speaks: Therapeutic dialogues for mind–body problems.* New York: Basic Books.

Groopman, J. (2007). *How doctors think.* Boston: Houghton Mifflin.

Gross, J. J. (Ed.). (2007). *Handbook of emotion regulation.* New York: Guilford Press.

Grunebaum, H. (1988). What if family therapy were a kind of psychotherapy?: A reading of the handbook of psychology and behavioral change. *Journal of Marital and Family Therapy, 14*(2), 195–199.

Gupta, M., Coyne, J. D., & Beach, S. R. H. (2003). Couples treatment for major depression: Critique of the literature and suggestions for some different directions. *Journal of Family Therapy, 25,* 317–346.

Gurman, A. S. (2002). Brief integrative marital therapy: A depth-behavioral approach. In A. S. Gurman & N. S. Jacobson (Eds.), *Clinical handbook of couple therapy* (3rd ed., pp. 180–220). New York: Guilford Press.

Halford, W. K., Markman, H. J., Kline, G. H., & Stanley, S. M. (2003). Best practice in couple relationship education. *Journal of Marital and Family Therapy, 29,* 385–406.

Henggeler, S. W., Pickrel, S. G., & Brodino, M. J. (1999). Multisystemic treatment of substance abusing and dependent delinquents: Outcomes, treatment fidelity, and transportability. *Mental Health Services Research, 1*(3), 171–184.

Henline, B., & Howard, M. (2008). Understanding and treating cyber-betrayal. *Family Therapy, 7*(2), 25–29.

Hetherington, E. M., & Stanley-Hagan, M. (2002). Parenting in divorced and remarried families. In M. Bornstein (Ed.), *Handbook of parenting* (2nd ed., pp. 287–316). Mahwah, NJ: Erlbaum.

Hirschfeld, R., & Russell, J. (1997). Assessment and treatment of suicidal patients. *New England Journal of Medicine, 337*(13), 910–915.

Hof, L., & Berman, E. (1986). The sexual genogram. *Journal of Marital and Family Therapy, 12,* 39–47.

Hoffman, L. (1981). *Foundations of family therapy.* New York: Basic Books.

Hofstra, M., Van der Ende, J., & Verhulst, F. (2000, July). Continuity and change of psychopathology from childhood into adulthood: A 14-year follow-up study. *Journal of the American Academy of Child and Adolescent Psychiatry, 39*(7), 850–858.

Hunsley, J., & Mash, E. (2005). Developing guidelines for the evidence-based assessment of adult disorders. *Psychological Assessment, 17,* 251–255.

Imber-Black, E. (1988). *Families and larger systems: A family therapist's guide through the labyrinth.* New York: Guilford Press.

Insel, T. R., & Quirion, R. (2005). Psychiatry as a clinical neuroscience discipline. *Journal of the American Medical Association, 294*(17), 2221–2224.

Integrated primary care: The central piece in the health care puzzle. (n.d.) Retrieved September 12, 2008, from *www.integratedprimarycare.com.*

Jacobson, N. S., & Gurman, A. S. (Eds.). (1995). *Clinical handbook of couple therapy.* New York: Guilford Press.

James, K., & McIntyre, D. (1983). The reproduction of families: The social role of the family. *Journal of Marital and Family Therapy, 9,* 119–129.

Johnson, S. (2004). *The practice of emotionally focused couple therapy: Creating connection.* New York: Brunner-Routledge.

Kase, L., & Ledley, D. R. (2007). *Anxiety disorders.* Hoboken, NJ: Wiley.

Kaslow, F. (2000). Families experiencing divorce. In W. C. Nichols, M. A. Pace-Nichols, D. S. Becvar, & A. Y Napier (Eds.), *Handbook of family development and intervention* (pp. 341–368). New York: Wiley.

Kazdin, A. E. (1997). Parent-management training: Evidence, outcomes, and issues. *Journal of the American Academy of Child and Adolescent Psychiatry, 36,* 1349–1356.

Keeling, M. L., & Piercy, F. P. (2007). A careful balance: Multinational perspectives on culture, gender, and power in marriage and family therapy practice. *Journal of Marital and Family Therapy, 33*(4), 443–463.

Keitner, G., Ryan, C., Miller, I., & Kohn, R. (1993). The role of the family in major depressive illness. *Psychiatric Annals, 23*(9), 500–507.

Kessler, R., Adler, L., Barkley, R., Biederman, J., Conners, K., Demler, O., et al. (2006). The prevalence and correlates of adult ADHD in the United States: Results from the national comorbidity survey replication. *Archives of General Psychiatry, 163*(4), 716–722.

Kessler, R., Berglund, P., Demler, O., Jin, R., Merikangas, K. R., & Walters, E. E. (2005). Lifetime prevalence and age-of-onset distributions of DSM-IV disorders in the National Comorbidity Survey replication. *Archives of General Psychiatry, 62*(6), 593–602.

Kessler, R., Chiu, W. T., Demler, O., & Walters, E. E. (2005). Prevalence, severity, and comorbidity of 12-month DSM-IV disorders in the national comorbidity survey replication. *Archives of General Psychiatry, 62,* 617–627.

Kessler, R., Eaton, W., Wittchen, H., & Zhao, S. (1994). DSM-III-R: Generalized anxiety disorder in the national comorbidity survey. *Archives of General Psychiatry, 51*(5), 355–364.

Kitchens, J. M. (1994). Does this patient have an alcohol problem? *Journal of the American Medical Association, 272*(22), 1782–1787.

Kung, W. W. (2000). The intertwined relationship between depression and marital distress: Elements of marital therapy conducive to effective treatment outcome. *Journal of Marital and Family Therapy, 26,* 51–63.

Lawson, A. (1989). *Adultery: An analysis of love and betrayal.* New York: Basic Books.

Lebow, J. (2004). The integrative revolution in couple and family therapy. *Family Process, 36,* 1–17.

Liddle, H., & Dakof, G. (1995). Efficacy of family therapy for drug abuse: Promising but not definitive. *Journal of Marital and Family Therapy, 21*(4), 511–543.

Liddle, H. A. (1992). Family psychology: Progress and prospects of a maturing discipline. *Journal of Family Psychology, 5*(3–4), 249–263.

Liddle, H. A. (1999). Theory development in a family-based therapy for adolescent drug abuse. *Journal of Clinical Child Psychology, 28,* 521–532.

Lindblad-Goldberg, M. (1989). Successful minority single-parent families. In L. Combrinck-Graham (Ed.), *Children in family contexts* (pp. 116–134). New York: Guilford Press.

Livingston, S., & Bowen, L. (2006). Treating divorce families in family therapy: A literature review. In C. A. Everett & R. E. Lee (Eds.), *When marriages fail: Systemic family therapy interventions and issues* (pp. 3–20). New York: Haworth Press.

Locke, H. J., & Wallace, K. M. (1959). Short term marital adjustment and prediction tests: Their reliability and validity. *Journal of Marriage and Family Living, 21,* 251–255.

MacFarlane, M. (2003). Systemic treatment of depression: An integrative approach. *Journal of Family Psychotherapy, 14*(1), 43–61.

Margulies, S. (2007). *Working with divorcing spouses: How to help clients navigate the emotional and legal minefield.* New York: Guilford Press.

Markman, H. J., Stanley, S. M., & Blumberg, S. L. (2001). *Fighting for your marriage: Positive steps for preventing divorce and preserving a lasting love* (rev. ed.). San Francisco: Jossey-Bass.

Mash, E., & Hunsley, J. (2005). Evidence-based assessment of child and adolescent disorders: Issues and challenges. *Journal of Clinical Child and Adolescent Psychology, 34,* 362–379.

McCollum, E. E. (1990). Integrating structural-strategic and Bowen approaches in training beginning family therapists. *Contemporary Family Therapy, 12,* 23–34.

McGoldrick, M., & Carter, B. (2003). The family life cycle. In F. Walsh (Ed.), *Normal family processes: Growing diversity and complexity* (3rd ed., pp. 375–398). New York: Guilford Press.

McGoldrick, M., Gerson, R., & Petri, S. (2008). *Genograms: Assessment and intervention* (3rd ed.). New York: Norton.

McGrath, E., Keita, G. P., Strickland, B. R., & Russon, N. F. (1990). *Women and depression: Risk factors and treatment issues.* Washington, DC: American Psychological Association.

McLean, P., Miller, L., McLean, C., Chodkiewicz, A., & Whittal, M. (2006). Integrating psychological and biological approaches to anxiety disorders: Best practices within a family context. *Journal of Family Psychotherapy, 17*(3), 7–34.

McNeil, B. J. (2001). Hidden barriers to improvement in the quality of care. *New England Journal of Medicine, 345*(22), 1612–1620.

Miklowitz, D. J. (2008). *Bipolar disorder: A family-focused treatment approach* (2nd ed.). New York: Guilford Press.

Miller, S., & Sherrard, P. A. D. (1999). Couple communication: A system for equipping partners to talk, listen, and resolve conflicts effectively. In R. Berger & M. T. Hannah (Eds.), *Preventive approaches in couples therapy* (pp. 73–105). Philadelphia: Brunner/Mazel.

Miller, S. D., Duncan, B. L., & Hubble, M. A. (1997). *Escape from Babel: Toward a unifying language for psychotherapy practice.* New York: Norton.

Miller, W., & Rollnick, S. (2002). *Motivational interviewing: Preparing people for change.* New York: Guilford Press.

Minuchin, P., Colapinto, J., & Minuchin, S. (2006). *Working with families of the poor* (2nd ed.). New York: Guilford Press.

Minuchin, S. (1974). *Families and family therapy.* Cambridge, MA: Harvard University Press.

Minuchin, S., & Fishman, H. C. (1981). *Family therapy techniques.* Cambridge, MA: Harvard University Press.

Minuchin, S., Montalvo, B., Guerney, B. G., Rosman B. L., & Schumer, F. (1967). *Families of the slums.* New York: Basic Books.

Mohr, D., Vella, L., Hart, S., Heckman, T., & Simon, G. (2008). The effect of telephone-administered psychotherapy on symptoms of depression and attrition: A meta-analysis. *Clinical Psychology: Science and Practice, 15*(3), 243–253.

Moltz, D. (1993). Bipolar disorder and the family: An integrative model. *Family Process, 32*(4), 409–423.

Morris, T. L., & March, J. S. (Eds.). (2004). *Anxiety disorders in children and adolescents* (2nd ed.). New York: Guilford Press.

Napier, A. Y., & Whitaker, C. (1978). *The family crucible.* New York: Harper & Row.

National Conference of Commissioners on Uniform State Laws. (1970). *Uniform Marriage and Divorce Act.* Chicago: Author. (Approved by the American Bar Association in 1974.)

Nichols, M. P., & Schwartz, R. C. (2007). *Family therapy: Concepts and methods.* New York: Allyn & Bacon.

Nichols, W. C. (1988). *Marital therapy: An integrative approach.* New York: Guilford Press.

Nichols, W. C., & Everett, C. A. (1986). *Systemic family therapy.* New York: Guilford Press.

Norcross, J. C., & Guy, J. D. (2007). *Leaving it at the office: A guide to psycho-therapist self-care.* New York: Guilford Press.

Northey, W. (2002). Characteristics and clinical practices of marriage and family therapists: A national survey. *Journal of Marital and Family Therapy, 28*(4), 487–494.

Northey, W. F., Wells, K. C., Silverman, W. K., & Bailey, C. E. (2003). Childhood behavioral and emotional disorders. *Journal of Marital and Family Therapy, 29,* 523–546.

O'Brian, C., & Bruggen, P. (1985). Our personal and professional lives: Learning positive connotation and circular questions. *Family Process, 24,* 311–322.

O'Farrell, T. J., & Fals-Stewart, W. (2006). Behavioral couples therapy for alcoholism and drug abuse. New York: Guilford Press.

Ogrodniczuk, J. S., Joyce, A. S., & Piper, W. E. (2005). Strategies for reducing patient-initiated premature termination of psychotherapy. *Harvard Review of Psychiatry, 13*(2), 57–70.

O'Hanlon, W. (1982). Strategic pattern intervention. *Journal of Strategic and Systemic Therapies, 4,* 26–33.

Pallanti, S. (2006). From impulse-control disorders toward behavioral addictions. *CNS Spectrums, 11*(12), 921–922.

Paolucci, E. O., Genius, M. L., & Violato, C. (2001). A meta-analysis of the published research on the effects of child sexual abuse. *Journal of Psychology, 135*(1), 17–36.

Papernow, P. L. (1993). *Becoming a stepfamily.* San Francisco: Jossey-Bass.

Pasley, K., Rhoden, L., Visher, E. B., and Visher, J. S. (1996). Successful stepfamily therapy: Clients' perspectives. *Journal of Marital and Family Therapy, 22,* 342–357.

Patterson, J. E., Albala, A. A., MacCahill, M. E., & Edwards, T. M. (2006). *The therapist's guide to psychopharmacology: Working with patients, families, and physicians to optimize care.* New York: Guilford Press.

Patterson, J. E., & Magulac, M. (1994). The family therapist's guide to psychopharmacology: A graduate level course. *Journal of Marital and Family Therapy, 20*(2), 151–173.

Patterson, J., Miller, R., Carnes, S., & Wilson, S. (2007). Evidence-based practice for marriage and family therapists. *Journal of Marital and Family Therapy, 30,* 183–195.

Penn, C. D., Hernandez, S. L., & Bermudez, J. M. (1997). Using a cross-cultural perspective to understand infidelity in couples therapy. *American Journal of Family Therapy, 25,* 169–185.

Pfeiffer, E. (1975). A short portable mental status questionnaire for the assessment of organic brain deficit in elderly patients. *Journal of the American Geriatric Society, 23,* 433–441.

Prince, S., & Jacobson, N. (1995). Couple and family therapy for depression. In E. E. Beckham & W. R. Leber (Eds.), *Handbook of depression* (2nd ed., pp. 404–424). New York: Guilford Press.

Prochaska, J., Norcross, J., & DiClemente, C. (1994). *Changing for good.* New York: Avon.

Rapee, R., Wignall, A., Spence, S., Cobham, V., & Lyneham, H. (2008). *Helping your anxious child*. Oakland, CA: New Harbinger.

Rappaport, L. (1970). Crisis intervention as a brief mode of treatment. In R. W. Roberts & R. H. Nee (Eds.), *Theories of social casework* (pp. 123–159). Chicago: University of Chicago Press.

Renk, K., & Dinger, T. M. (2002). Reasons for therapy termination in a university psychology clinic. *Journal of Clinical Psychology, 58*, 1173–1181.

Riggs, D. S., Caulfield, M. B., & Street, A. E. (2000). Risk for domestic violence: Factors associated with perpetration and victimization. *Journal of Clinical Psychology, 56*, 1289–1316.

Rogers, C. R. (1972). *On becoming a person*. Boston: Houghton Mifflin.

Rowe, C. L., & Liddle, H. A. (2007). Substance abuse. *Journal of Marital and Family Therapy, 29*(1), 97–120.

Rumstein-McKean, O., & Hunsley, J. (2001). Interpersonal and family functioning of female survivors of childhood sexual abuse. *Clinical Psychology Review, 21*, 471–490.

Sackett, D. L., Strauss, S., Richardson, S. W., Rosenberg, W., & Haynes, B. R. (2000). *Evidence-based medicine: How to practice and teach EBM*. New York: Churchill Livingstone.

Sapolsky, R. (2005). *Monkeyluv*. New York: Scribner.

Satir, V. (1967). *Conjoint family therapy*. Palo Alto, CA: Science & Behavior Books.

Saunders, J. B., Aasland, O. G., Babor, T. F., De La Fuente, J. R., & Grant, M. (1993). Development of the Alcohol Use Disorders Identification Test (AUDIT): WHO collaborative project on early detection of persons with harmful alcohol consumption (II). *Addiction, 88*, 791–804.

Schore, A. (2003a). *Affect dysregulation and disorders of the self*. New York: Norton.

Schore, A. (2003b). *Affect regulation and the repair of the self*. New York: Norton.

Schore, A. (2005). Back to basics: Attachment, affect regulation, and the right brain: Linking developmental neuroscience to pediatrics. *Pediatrics in Review, 26*(6), 204–217.

Seaburn, D., Landau-Stanton, J., & Horwitz, S. (1995). Core techniques in family therapy. In R. H. Mikesell, D. Lusterman, & S. H. McDaniel (Eds.), *Integrating family therapy: Handbook of family psychology and systems theory* (pp. 5–26). Washington, DC: American Psychological Association.

Selzer, M. L. (1971). The Michigan Alcoholism Screening Test: The quest for a new diagnostic instrument. *American Journal of Psychiatry, 127*, 1653–1658.

Sexton, T. L., Sydnor, A. E., Rowland, M. K., & Alexander, J. F. (2005). Behavioral and relationship problems. In R. H. Coombs (Ed.), *Family therapy review: Preparing for comprehensive and licensing examinations* (pp. 349–370). Mahwah, NJ: Erlbaum.

Shadish, W. R., & Baldwin, S. A. (2003). Meta-analysis of MFT interventions. *Journal of Marital and Family Therapy, 29*(4), 547–570.

Shaw, P., Eckstrand, K., Sharp, W., Blumenthal, J., Lerch, J. P., Greenstein, D., et al. (2007). Attention-deficit/hyperactivity disorder is characterized by a delay in cortical maturation. *Proceedings of the National Academy of Sciences of the United States of America, 104*(49), 19649–19654.

Shea, M. T., Gibbons, R., Elkin, I., & Sotsky, S. (1995). Initial severity and differential treatment outcome in the National Institute of Mental Health Treatment of Depression of Collaborative Research Program. *Journal of Consulting and Clinical Psychology, 63*(5), 841–847.

Shear, K., Frank, E., Houck, P. R., & Reynolds, C. F. (2005). Treatment of complicated grief: A randomized controlled trial. *Journal of the American Medical Association, 293*, 2601–2608.

Siegel, D. J. (1999). *The developing mind: How relationships and the brain interact to shape who we are.* New York: Guilford Press.

Siegel, D. J. (2007). *The mindful brain: Reflection and attunement in the cultivation of well-being.* New York: Norton.

Skovholt, T. M., & Rønnestad, M. H., & (2003). Struggles of the novice counselor and therapist. *Journal of Career Development, 30*, 45–58.

Snyder, D. K. (1979). Multidimensional assessment of marital satisfaction. *Journal of Marriage and Family, 41*(4), 813–823.

Snyder, D. K., Castellani, A. M., & Whisman, M. A. (2006). Current status and future directions in couple therapy. *Annual Review of Psychology, 57*, 317–344.

Spanier, G. B. (1976). Measuring marital adjustment: New scales for assessing the quality of marriage and similar dyads. *Journal of Marriage and Family, 38*, 15–28.

Sprenkle, D. H., & Bischoff, R. J. (1991). Research in family therapy: Trends, issues and recommendations. In M. Nichols & R. Schwartz (Eds.), *Family therapy: Concepts and methods* (pp. 542–580). Boston: Allyn & Bacon.

Sprenkle, D. H., & Blow, A. J. (2004). Common factors and our sacred models. *Journal of Marital and Family Therapy, 30*, 113–129.

Steinglass, P., Bennett, L. A., Wolin, S. J., & Reiss, D. (1987). *The alcoholic family.* New York: Basic Books.

Straus, M. A. (1979). Measuring intrafamily conflict and violence: The Conflict Tactics Scale. *Journal of Marriage and Family, 41*, 75–88.

Szapocznik, J., Perez-Vidae, A., Brickman, A. L., Foote, F. H., Santisteban, O., & Hervis, W. M. (1988). Engaging adolescent drug abusers and their families in treatment: A strategic structural systems approach. *Journal of Consulting and Clinical Psychology, 56*, 552–557.

Szapocznik, J., & Williams, R. A. (2000). Brief strategic family therapy: Twenty-five years of interplay among theory, research and practice in adolescent behavioral problems and abuse. *Clinical Child and Family Psychology Review, 3*, 117–135.

Taggart, M. (1985). The feminist critique in epistemological perspective: Questions of context in family therapy. *Journal of Marital and Family Therapy, 11*, 113–126.

Taylor, R. (1990). *Distinguishing psychological from organic disorders: Screening for psychological masquerades.* New York: Springer.

Tomm, K. (1988). Interventive interviewing: Part III. *Family Process, 27*(1), 1–15.

Treas, J., & Giesen, D. (2000). Sexual infidelity among married and cohabiting Americans. *Journal of Marriage and Family, 62*, 48–60.

Uebelacker, L., Weishaar, M., & Miller, I. (2008). Family or relationship problems. In M. A. Whisman (Ed.), *Adapting cognitive therapy for depression: Managing complexity and comorbidity* (pp. 326–347). New York: Guilford Press.

U.S. Census Bureau. (2000). Retrieved March 2009, from *www.census.gov. main/www/cen2000.html.*

Visher, E. B., & Visher, J. S. (1988). *Old loyalties, new ties: Therapeutic strategies with stepfamilies.* New York: Brunner/Mazel.

Visher, E. B., & Visher, J. S. (1996). *Therapy with stepfamilies.* New York: Brunner/Mazel.

Weber, T., & Levine, F. (1995). Engaging the family: An integrative approach. In R. H. Mikesell, D. Lusterman, & S. H. McDaniel (Eds.), *Integrating family therapy: Handbook of family psychology and systems theory* (pp. 45–72). Washington, DC: American Psychological Association.

Wechsler, D. (1991). *Wechsler Intelligence Scale for Children* (3rd ed.). San Antonio, TX: Psychological Corporation.

Weeks, G. R. (1989). *Treating couples: The intersystem model of the Marriage Council of Philadelphia.* New York: Brunner/Mazel.

Weeks, G. R., Odell, M., & Methven, S. (2005). *If only I had known . . . : Avoiding common mistakes in couples therapy.* New York: Norton.

Weiss, R., & Cerrato, M. (1980). The marital status inventory: Development of a measure of dissolution potential. *American Journal of Family Therapy, 8*(2), 80–85.

Williams, L., & Day, A. (2007). Strategies for dealing with clients we dislike. *American Journal of Family Therapy, 35*, 83–92.

Williams, L. M., Patterson, J., & Miller, R. B. (2006). Panning for gold: A clinician's guide to using research. *Journal of Marital and Family Therapy, 32*, 17–32.

Williams, L. M., & Winter, H. (2009). Guidelines for an effective transfer of cases: The needs of the transfer triad. *American Journal of Family Therapy, 37*, 146–158.

Wolf, E. S. (1988). *Treating the self: Elements of clinical self psychology.* New York: Guilford Press.

Yalom, I. D. (2002). *The gift of therapy: An open letter to a new generation of therapists and their patients.* New York: HarperCollins.

Index